INTRODUCTORY PSYCHOLOGY

Founded by C. K. Ogden

The International Library of Psychology

GENERAL PSYCHOLOGY
In 38 Volumes

INTRODUCTORY PSYCHOLOGY

An Approach For Social Workers

D R PRICE-WILLIAMS

First published in 1958 by
Routledge and Kegan Paul Ltd

Reprinted in 1999 by
Routledge

2 Park Square, Milton Park, Abingdon, Oxfordshire OX14 4RN

711 Third Avenue, New York, NY 10017

Transferred to Digital Printing 2006
First issued in paperback 2014

Routledge is an imprint of the Taylor and Francis Group, an informa company

British Library Cataloguing in Publication Data
A CIP catalogue record for this book
is available from the British Library

Introductory Psychology
ISBN 978-0-415-21038-6 (hbk)
ISBN 978-0-415-75803-1 (pbk)
General Psychology: 38 Volumes
ISBN 978-0-415-21129-1
The International Library of Psychology: 204 Volumes
ISBN 978-0-415-19132-6
Printed and bound by CPI Antony Rowe, Eastbourne

CONTENTS

PREFACE

THIS volume was originally designed as a text-book for students of Social Work. On being appointed to provide a course of lectures in Psychology for students taking the Certificate in Social Science and Administration, I was impressed by the lack of an adequate introductory text. Existing text-books, although I have gratefully leaned upon them here, did not appear to provide a balance of material appropriate to these students, and were mainly designed for those taking Psychology as a main subject. The decision was then taken to attempt a new approach. By extension, it was thought that the present volume might be suitable for social workers in general, and for those people whose studies bring them to the perimeter of Psychology without going the whole way. Accordingly this book is provided both as a framework and a foundation for such students. It does not go beyond elementary principles and it does not treat of specialist topics. It is designed as a bridge to specialised subjects, such as the Psychology of the Family, Marriage, Delinquency and so on. I also count Psycho-Analysis as a specialist subject, but some material has been given here. I would like to emphasise that the approach has been given width rather than depth, so that the student can base his subsequent reading within a comprehensive structure.

There are a great many people to whom I am indebted. First of all I would like to thank Professor R. M. Titmuss for his primary encouragement. I am very much indebted to Dr. H. T. Himmelweit for her constant advice and interest. I am most grateful to Dr. A. N. Oppenheim who carefully corrected a part of the book. On the Social Work side I would like to thank Mrs. K. F. McDougall for her helpful opinions; also Miss L. H. Bell for advice on some points. My thanks are also due to the Social Research Division of the London School of Economics and Political Science for financial assistance in circulating early on in the writing an experimental chapter. At which stage Miss F.

Mitchell and Miss M. P. Keenleyside gave me useful indications of the line to take.

I am especially indebted to Professor W. J. H. Sprott for giving me his valuable advice and opinion both during the writing of the book and after it was completed. Lastly I must thank my wife upon whose patient ear the clarity of the paragraphs was tested.

D.R.P-W.

London School of Economics and
Political Science.
April 1957

I

INTRODUCTION

WHAT is Psychology? The expression "every man is his own philosopher" can be applied with equal force to the subject of Psychology, a feature which introduces difficulties as well as stimulates interest. The difficulties stem from the fact that the study of experience and the way people behave is open both to the layman and the professional psychologist, but the way which each sets about the study is different. The successful business man, the magistrate, the custom officer, even the confidence trickster, may pride himself on being a "psychologist". By this he means that he professes to understand people and is able to assess their actions. And he may be very successful in doing this. But this faculty does not make the business man or magistrate a "professional" psychologist. The latter is a person who *systematically* studies the behaviour of people—and animals—and who tries to *explain* their behaviour in the same sort of way that the physicist explains the behaviour of physical objects or the physiologist explains the functioning of our bodies. Psychology can therefore be defined as the systematic study of behaviour.

SCOPE OF PSYCHOLOGY

"Behaviour" is a wide term; it embraces relatively large reactions, such as criminal conduct, to relatively small reactions, as response to a bright light. It also includes those elements of experience that can be referred to something observable. So it is that the scope of psychology is very wide. It can range from the testing of children in a clinic to fitting the man to a job in a factory; from studying people in groups to investigating the reason why people vote for certain political parties; from the study of interpersonal relationships to the testing of rats in mazes.

A

The relationship of theory and practice in psychology requires a brief comment. Part of the task of a psychologist is to construct theories that will help to bring many diverse facts under one specific generalisation, and from which predictions are also able to be made. It should be pointed out at once that there are very few generalisations in psychology that are comparable with the breadth possible in physics for example. Ohm's law in physics tells us about the mutual relationships of resistance, voltage and current in all, or nearly all conductors. As is well known Newton's law of gravitation embraced a wide range of phenomena from falling apples to the movement of planets in their orbits. While there are not laws of this stature in psychology, there are lesser generalised statements which have been found to be true under specified conditions in certain fields. However it would be true to say that as regards the complex behaviour of human beings we are far from being able to formulate *rational* theories with the same success that has been gained in the natural sciences. What have been gained with some success in psychology are *empirical* statements based upon the results of observation and experiment. As a result of this it is not possible to apply practice from theory with the same exactitude as is possible in some other sciences. To state this is not to detract from the scientific status of psychology; it is to specify with caution the particular level at which, on the whole, we are operating. It is particularly necessary to emphasise this as a preface to the theories and findings reported in the present volume, as they constitute statements formulated at different levels, from the results of laboratory investigations to large scale observations. While it is necessary, for the sake of content, to cast the net wide, we should not be led to suppose that the fish caught thereby are of equal validity.

Fields of Psychology. One way of describing the scope of psychology is by specifying what psychologists do, and for this we can turn to the different fields in which they operate, keeping in mind throughout the distinction of the theoretical and the practical.

In the medical and clinical spheres, the psychologist must be distinguished from the psychiatrist. The latter is a person who has first a medical degree and then proceeds to specialise in the field of abnormal psychology. He is concerned with the study and treatment of nervous and mental disorders. The psychologist who works with patients suffering from nervous and mental disorders, applies his knowledge to the application of intelligence and personality tests, but also performs valuable service in research which aids our knowledge of mental illness. He cannot, however, with the exception of some non-medical psychotherapists, do treatment in the same way as the psychiatrist. The clinical psychologist does not only work in mental hospitals; he is employed[1] in psychiatric out-patient clinics, neurosis units, institutions for mental defectives, rehabilitation centres and general hospitals. Apart from the diagnosis of intellectual, personality and social features of patients, he assists indirectly in the sphere of treatment by recommending on the strength of his tests the type of treatment most likely to succeed, and indicating the nature of the response to psychiatric treatment. He can also play the role of advisor in rehabilitation of patients. Psychologists are also employed in the Prison Service where testing procedures are again used.

Educational psychology consists of the diagnosis, treatment and prevention of conditions which hinder learning and general development. Educational psychologists generally work in child guidance clinics, which come under the school psychological service of local educational authorities. Here they are concerned with[2] the assessment of the child's personality, his intellectual assets and his attainments. They also are connected with the re-education, readjustment and retraining of problem children, and act as liaison officers between the clinic and the school. More generally they assist in the educational guidance of children, both normal and backward.

Occupational psychologists study the behaviour of people at work, in industry, business and in government services. The problems with which they are concerned are the selection of personnel, vocational guidance, improving psychological working conditions by various means, facilitating communication between workers and management, and more generally increasing effectiveness at work. Occupational psychology can be summarised in the two statements: "fitting the man to the job" and "fitting the job to the man".

Apart from these three main streams, psychologists are employed in market research, which can include the response to

[1] *Bulletin of the British Psychological Society.* 1955 No. 25.
[2] *op. cit.*

advertisements as well as the reaction to radio and television programmes. Racial and social problems create further advisory capacities for the social psychologist. Besides all these applied fields, the psychologist is engaged in research, either of theoretical or practical problems, in universities, clinics, factories and schools, and in such a study as town-planning.

HISTORICAL ORIGINS

It has been said that psychology has had a long past but a short history, meaning that although speculations about the psyche date back to antiquity, it is only comparatively recently, within the last hundred years, that psychology has flowered as an independent discipline. The progenitors of modern psychology are philosophy, physiology and medicine. While psychology is of course very much inter-related with these studies, it can be said to contain a body of knowledge independent of them. The emancipation from other disciplines came about with the rise of "schools" of psychology, a feature which, due largely to the importance placed on experiment—to be considered later—has now given way to an integration of approaches. The schools can be summarised under four headings.

Introspectionism. Influenced by the observationalist tradition of the British empirical philosophers[3] there arose a school of thought at Würzburg which sought to make a classification of the contents of experience. It was thought, that by suitable training, observers could report on the very content of consciousness; that by paying attention to the "how" as well as to the "what" of thought, an inventory of the mind could be made. It was thought that sensations, feelings and images were the basic elements out of which complex mental events were made. The scheme envisaged was that of a collection of "mental bricks" out of which was made a "mental brick wall". Introspection as a systematic method of enquiry has now been largely discarded. It persists in the study of protocols of patients and as an indicative adjunct to what can be found out by other methods of research on people. However the Würzburg school did bring out the important fact that the mind was not a static entity, composed of little mental bricks, but was

[3] See Chapter 15 of Peters, R. S. (ed.) *Brett's History of Psychology*. Allen and Unwin, 1953.

4

composed of attitudes and tendencies which could not be reduced to sensations and images.

Behaviourism. Partly as a result of the impact of Darwin and partly as a result of the sterility which the introspective approach had engendered, there arose a school of thought which proclaimed that consciousness was but a sequence of automatic actions and that all that should be studied was the way in which a person behaved. In its extreme form behaviourism was no doubt, as Professor Broad once characterised it, a "silly" doctrine, but it did introduce reliability into psychological investigation. How a person behaves is a more reliable index than what he reports verbally. The latter method suffers from the detriment that what is experienced is private property; the actions of a person are at least public property. There can be common agreement as to what a person *does*. Because of the objectivity which this approach gave, psychologists paid more attention to phenomena which were amenable to objective observation and experiment. And while the term "behaviour" is considerably more elastic now than "behaviourism" in giving due place to unobservables, the principle has set in that psychology should pay close attention to verification.

Purposive Psychology. The introspection school had pictured the concept of mind as a static collection of elements. Behaviourism, while rejecting mind, had put forward a scheme of associative elements within a framework of stimulus and response. The school of purposive psychology, associated with the name of William McDougall, now put forward a dynamic psychology. Behaviour was not just a matter of a chain of automatic elements responding to a stimulus; it was purposive. Purposive striving was put forward as a principle of behaviour in place of the mechanistic picture painted by the behaviourist. Central to this viewpoint was the part played by instinct, a theme which we will discuss in Chapter II. Although McDougall's use of the word "purpose" was not altogether clear, this school of thought had its effect in directing the attention of psychologists to the "goal-seeking" aspects of behaviour, and provided a necessary counter to the extreme formulations of the behaviourist.[4] Modern

4 For an account of purposive or "hormic" psychology see Part IV Chapter VII of Flugel, J. C. *A Hundred Years of Psychology*. Duckworth 1951.

"neobehaviourism" can be said to be a synthesis of the purposive and behaviouristic approaches.

Psycho-Analysis. In Chapter VI we shall deal with the model of the personality revealed by the school of psycho-analysis, and from time to time throughout this book we shall refer to other aspects of it. It is perhaps necessary to note that the term strictly speaking pertains to the doctrines of Sigmund Freud, while the term "analytical psychology" refers to the school associated with C. G. Jung. Psycho-analysis is at once a technique and a doctrine. It arose from interpretations of clinical observations. From a study of his patients Freud was struck by the fact that there were certain mental factors which influenced their experience and behaviour, although they were not aware of them. These factors were in fact *unconscious*. An investigation of these unconscious factors produced a body of theories which we shall discuss later. It is to be noted that the psycho-analytic approach also put forward a dynamic picture of the mind, opposed to behaviourism, while its emphasis on the unconscious has marked it off from other approaches. It is also to be noted that the technique and the theories go hand in hand. The technique is a method of treating mental illness, by primarily psychological methods (to be described later in the book) as distinct from physical or chemical methods. The theories of psycho-analysis have evolved from the use of the technique. While many of Freud's findings have been corroborated by other methods of enquiry, many others can be tested only *via* the technique itself.

There remains another school of psychology which had a great influence, namely the Gestalt school, but we shall consider the ideas belonging to this approach in the chapter on Perception.

THE RISE OF SCIENTIFIC METHOD

It has become natural for the psychologist to put his assumptions about human nature to the same sort of testing procedure as the natural scientist does with assumptions about the world of inanimate things. The assumption that balls of different weight fall at the same rate remains a supposition until it is put to the test. For centuries in fact the reverse was believed to be true, and it was not until it was put to the experimental test, until in fact somebody actually systematically dropped balls of different weights and observed their rate of falling, was the old assumption exploded. Similarly in psychology speculations remain speculations until they can be put to the test of experiment or observation.

Experimentation. What are the requirements of a scientific experiment? We mentioned the testing of falling bodies. Here there were two important elements: the different weights of the balls and the time they took to fall to the ground. The factor varied was weight, the response was the time taken to fall. In technical language these two elements of an experiment are known as the *independent* and *dependent variable* respectively. The independent variable is the factor manipulated by the experimenter, the dependent variable is the response. To take a psychological example: if we wished to know the effects on production in a factory of a "Music while you work" programme, the experiment would be made by relaying the broadcast while the workers were carrying on with their jobs. The programme constitutes the independent variable, the production rates of the workers represent the dependent variable. However the situation is seldom as simple as this. If an independent variable is to be tested for its consequences then extraneous factors have to be kept out of the way. To refer back to the experiment with the balls. If the falling of the balls was timed separately, then the conditions under which the experiment was made would have to be similar. Otherwise there might occur an outside factor such as a high wind when one ball was dropped, which would upset the experiment. In the music while you work experiment, two extraneous factors might be operative. It could be that the production of those workers was ascending at that time anyhow, and therefore had nothing to do with the programme. Or it could be that it was not the music that altered the production, but merely the fact that there was some noise going on.

These difficulties point to the necessity of *control*. We must be sure that the particular result that we gain from an experiment is dependent on the factor that we are manipulating. One way of surmounting the first difficulty with the factory workers would be to compare production rates with no programme over a period of time, with the production rates with programmes introduced at odd moments over a period of months. The two conditions could then be compared with justification, always assuming that there was not some other influence appearing at exactly the same time as the programme. With the second difficulty, that the workers were not responding to the music so much as to the noise, a control situation could be introduced by alternating the music programme with a talk, and comparing the two results.

A control situation can be made with individuals or with groups. A *"control group"* is a common feature in psychological experimentation. If one wishes to see if a reward has the effect of accelerating the learning of a task with a group of schoolboys, it is necessary to compare this group with a control group of boys who do the same task but gain no reward. This leads to the condition known as *matching*. If one wishes to compare the performances of two groups of boys as in the above case, ideally we would like to know that they both have similar characteristics. Otherwise it might happen that the "reward" group was composed of boys of quick intelligence, and the "control no-reward" group was a bunch of dullards. Prior to the experiment therefore a matching procedure would have to be done, so that the two groups were about equal in intelligence. The relevant factors in such an experiment must always be matched.

Systematic Observation. Obviously not all factors of psychological interest can be experimentally investigated, nor need they call for the use of experiment. The emotional development of children, for example, can be studied systematically by observing the behaviour of children over many years. Observation, however, does entail selection. We cannot observe everything, and we select those items which we consider to be important. Observation is not wholly independent of the principles of experimentation. Control methods can be used. If we wish to observe the effects of television on people's habits, then there is required for the sake of assessment, two different groups, the viewers and the non-viewers. These, further, will have to be matched for age, intelligence, social class and other variables which are deemed to be of importance. Observation, therefore, is not simply a matter of "having a look"; it requires prior planning and arrangement.

Statistics. Modern statistical methods are useful tools for analysing complicated psychological features. We cannot discuss the various methods used in psychology[5], but it is necessary to define one or two terms that will be used throughout the text.

If we take measurements of a variable among a large number of cases, let us say those of the heights of boys in a school, there are three basic measurements that can be ascertained. The first is the *mean* or average. It is merely the sum of all the different heights divided by the number of boys. The actual figure calculated may not correspond to any individual boy's height. The mean height of four boys of four, four, five and six feet respectively is nineteen divided by four, which comes to four and three-quarters feet. The *mode* is the figure which occurs most frequently. In a large number of boys it could be that four feet six inches was the height that occurred most frequently, although this need not be the mean. The *median* score is the middlemost one. If we lined up five boys along a wall in order of increasing height, the height of the third boy would represent the median score. Again this need not be the mean. In cases where the distribution of any variable is normal, the three measures of central tendency will be identical.

The mean gives us important information about a number of cases. But we generally wish to know more about the *distribution* of a variable. Particularly we would like to know about the range of measurements around the mean. It could happen that in two sets of cases the mean is identical, but that the individual scores about the mean in each set is very different. For example, five boys might produce scores in an intelligence test of 100, 101, 102, 103, 104 respectively. The mean here is the score of the middlemost boy, namely 102 (note that in this case the mean equals the median). On the other hand we might have another set of five boys whose scores range in the following sequence: 50, 90, 100, 120, 150. Here again the mean is 102. Plainly, although the mean of each set is identical, the two groups are widely divergent. In the first case the individual scores are all very close to the average, while in the second case they are widely scattered. Were we to rely solely on the mean for an indication of the boys' performances our conclusions would be very wrong. We need some measure in order to allow for this kind of difference. An important measure that is used for indicating such a dispersion is the *standard deviation*. It is calculated by finding the squares of each individual difference

[5] A useful book which contains some psychological examples is Moroney, M. J. *Facts from Figures.* Pelican Books 1953

from the mean, dividing the sum of these by the number of cases, and taking the square root of the total. The figure calculated gives us new information about the "shape" of the scores of the group tested. Without going into the exact calculations necessary in the above example, it is easy to visualise that the form of the curve plotted to depict the distribution of the individual scores is narrow in the first case and wide in the second.

An important statistical term that we shall use often is *correlation*. In psychology it is very often the case, as in other sciences, that we have two series of measurements that appear to have some connection with each other. The variations of atmospheric pressure varies concomitantly with the variations of mercury in a tube. The fluctuations of interest in a cinema audience has some connection with the different events portrayed on the screen. In many cases we want to know the amount of correlation, whether there is in fact a connection between this phenomenon and that, whether it is positive or whether it is negative. For example three brothers may come out in the order of first, second, third, consistently in their school subjects of arithmetic, languages, and handicraft. We then say that as far as these three subjects are concerned there is a *positive* correlation between the boys' performances. The order of the boys is always similar in all their subjects. On the other hand if it should turn out that a boy who regularly came top in Latin, also came regularly bottom in Geometry, we should speak of a *negative* correlation, meaning that there would seem to be some connection between his being good at classics but bad at mathematics. There are statistical methods which calculate accurately the amount of correlation. The measurement of correlation runs from plus one which marks off perfect positive correlation through zero to minus one which represents perfect negative correlation. Zero correlation means that there is no connection at all; if one correlated the length of people's noses with their intelligence, the result would neither be positive nor negative. The connection is meaningless, and the correlation would be zero. This measure does not mean that the one series of measurements is the *cause* of the other, but it offers an indication that there is some probable connection between the two phenomena measured. Thus if we know that the correlation between tested intelligence and length of schooling is plus ·8, say, then we have grounds for belief that the two are connected in a causal way.

This is an obvious case, but there are other instances in which a connection is not so obvious, and here the measure of correlation can assist.

The following chapters contain material culled both from experimental enquiry and from naturalistic observation. Starting from a consideration of those factors that prompt people to action, we turn to the mechanisms that influence our knowledge and awareness of the world and of ourselves. In Chapter V the way in which this knowledge and awareness is transmitted to others is considered, while in the final chapter the total personality is discussed from different standpoints.

II

MOTIVATION

In daily life there is found an abundance of actions performed by people which makes it necessary to posit some underlying mechanism in order to account for them. One man stays at home and builds up a vast collection of British Colonial stamps, another travels to the Himalayas and ascends a hitherto unconquered peak. Schliemann from a very early age had the ambition to discover the ancient site of Troy; Amundsen longed to be a polar explorer since adolescence. While some people have relatively simple desires such as the satisfaction of bodily impulses, others are compelled by a dynamic restlessness to break the world record in pole-squatting. In short, different people have different wants and they perform various actions in order to satisfy them. The study of these different wants is the study of motivation.

CLASSIFICATION

There has been no lack of ways of describing motivation in the history of thought, although the word itself may not have been invoked. Whether it has been in the guise of desires, passions, impulses, wishes, aspirations, aims or drives, the concept has been used from the earliest times. The employment of different terms to explain the same mechanism has led to an inevitable confusion of terminology, and it is often only possible to define accurately some of these terms by relating them to the context, whether historical or experimental.

A somewhat rough classification of motives can be reached by separating the demands of the body from the demands aroused by interaction with people. In other words one can separate physiological determinants, such as hunger and thirst and sex, from acquired motives, such as the desire for wealth and power, the need for social acceptance, and some forms of fear. Acquired motives, therefore, do not arise from the way in which our bodies are organised, but are formed through the experience of a person, especially during the early formative years.

Motivation is a general term; there are a number of subsidiary terms within the general heading which require definition.

Need refers to a lack of something within the individual which requires to be filled. This may be of an organic nature, such as the need for food in hunger or the need for water in thirst, or it can be more of an acquired type such as need for approval.

Drive is similar to need, but it has the added criterion in that it is generally defined in terms of the goal to be reached. Thus we speak of the hunger drive, the sex drive and so forth. Although it is possible to speak of acquired drives, the term generally has a physiological meaning. The term *motive* itself can be kept for the more personal and social types of motivation.

Incentive is used as the end result of an activity, the goal to be attained.

If we use the familiar picture of the carrot which prompts the donkey, we can say that the animal has a need for food, which results in it being driven in search of the carrot, which is the incentive or goal. The sequence can be looked upon as a cycle, in which the attainment of the last stage, the reaching of the goal, satisfies the need which is the first stage.

INSTINCT

This term refers to the fact that there is a factor or set of factors inherent in man and animals that causes a sequence of actions to appear in the animal's lifetime, and which, as far as can be seen, is not learned or acquired by experience. The construction of a web by a spider is a facility which this creature has not learned from other spiders; it is a sequence of behaviour which is inherent in the spider organism. It is innate and not learned. Similarly certain bird songs are innate and not learned, as is easily demonstrated by rearing a bird in isolation so that it cannot hear the characteristic notes from other members of its species. When there is such a demonstration as this, and we can be quite certain that no element of experience has entered, we can be quite justified in labelling the singing as instinctive. Unfortunately human beings cannot be so experimentally treated, so that when the term is applied to man there is not such a precise meaning. Psychologists have differed in the past as to the number of instincts claimed for man. William James[1] listed several dozen instincts in man. McDougall[2] postulated at first seven major instincts. He defined the term as "an inherited or innate psycho-physical disposition which determines its possessor to perceive or pay attention to objects of a certain class, to experience an emotional excitement of a particular quality upon perceiving such an object, and to act in a particular manner or at least to experience an impulse to such action." Each major instinct was accompanied by a characteristic emotion. The instincts and their emotional tone were: escape (fear), repulsion (disgust), curiosity (wonder), pugnacity (anger), self-assertion (elation), self-abasement (subjection) and parental (tender emotion). These instincts are only of a historical importance, because a later list by McDougall extended the list to fourteen, and subsequently[3] he dropped the term altogether and postulated instead eighteen "propensities" and several "abilities".

These are relatively early speculations. At a more recent date the status of the term can be guessed by the title of the symposium "Is the Doctrine of Instincts Dead?"[4] Yet the matter still has its practical side because as Sir Cyril Burt has pointed out, if the contention is correct that the primitive instincts inherited from our animal ancestors form the basis of character and the most common source of juvenile crime, then any theory of character-training should be based upon an acceptable theory of instincts. It should be added that this viewpoint was not held by another contributor to the symposium, who maintained, on the contrary, that instincts were of no great interest to the practical psychologist or the teacher.

It is difficult to resolve these two opposing views. What is apparent is that although instinctive behaviour is clearly observable in some infra-human activities, when we come to such a complex organism as man it is difficult to separate that which is innately determined from that which is acquired, particularly so when there has been very early training.

---

[1] James, William. *Principles of Psychology.* 1890.
[2] McDougall, W. *An Introduction to Social Psychology.* 1908.
[3] McDougall, W. *The Energies of Men.* 1932.
[4] *Brit. Journal of Educational Psychol.* 1941–43. Vols. 11–13.

HOMEOSTASIS

It has been found that many internal processes of the body consist of steady states which are maintained relatively independent of the fluctuations of the environment. The internal body temperature of mammals is an example. The concentration of glucose in the blood is another. These are constants which, in addition to being free from chance influences in the outside world, are restored to their steady state if disturbed from their initial balance. The term "homeostasis" was coined as a principle of generalisation of a number of such instances. The strict meaning of the term is applicable only to the internal chemical states of the organism, but in recent years the principle has been extended to include the behaviour of the external parts of the body and even intellectual processes.[5]

Homeostasis and Motivation. In relation to motivation the homeostatic argument is that man has certain biological constancies, which if lacking or disorientated, provoke a behaviour which sets out to restore the balance. In a simple way this can be understood in the example of an animal which under the stress of thirst searches for water. The internal mechanism of water balance becomes disturbed. This sets up a further mechanism—the one regulating movement—which enables the animal to walk to a supply of water and thus restore the balance. In more complex activities the method involved can be more circumnavigatory, but the mechanism is the same, namely to restore the basic process. It can be seen that this formulation fits in well with the terms of need, drive and incentive or goal which have been previously described. The needs of an organism are represented as steady states which when disturbed set up drives which are directed towards the goals which satisfy the needs and restore the balance.[6]

SOCIAL MOTIVES

The type of motivation that we are now considering is reflected in that class of behaviour stimulated by the interaction of people in society. The fact that man does not live in isolation arouses

[5] Dempsey, E. W. "Homeostasis". in Stevens, S. S. *Handbook of Experimental Psychology*. Wiley. 1951.
[6] Mace, C. A. "Homeostasis, Needs and Values". *Brit. J. Psychol.* 1953, *44*, 200.

in him impulses which involve other people and affect the society in which he lives. In this section we shall focus attention on those impulses which exercise the interests of the social worker and people involved in similar activities.

POWER AND DOMINANCE

Philosophers have discussed the influence of power in the lives of men as being a strong and dominant force. Thomas Hobbes writing in 1651 spoke of a "perpetual and restless desire of Power after power, that ceaseth only in death", while Bertrand Russell in his book called *Power* nearly three centuries later drew attention to the fact that the love of power is a characteristic of men who are causally important, as they have influence on the course of events. It is not the desire of power in a political sense that is solely of psychological importance. It is not only the Napoleons and Hitlers that call for analysis. In a lesser degree most people exhibit a modicum of power, whether it is merely a desire for ascendance over a marital partner or the urge to become a head of a business.

Social Dynamics. The social dynamics of power is a theme which has occupied the attention of many social psychologists, who were interested both in the inter-personal relationships of those involved and in the structure of the situation. An investigation[7] made on groups of boys living in cabins indicated that the awareness of power as a social force was prominent. The boys themselves perceived quite clearly whether or not a single member of their group had social power. The children defined this social power as the ability "to get others to do what he wants them to". This awareness of power in others, or as the authors called it "attributed power", had a considerable generalisation. That is to say if a certain boy had achieved some eminence in sports, for example, his dominance in this sphere was generalised to all the activities of the group. The inter-relationship of these boys was influenced by the struggle for dominance. That this particular motive is at least partly dependent on the prevailing social climate was demonstrated in another study made with children.[8] In this

[7] Lippitt, R., Polansky, N,. and Rosen, S. "The Dynamics of Power". *Human Relations* 1952, *5*, 37.

[8] McCandless, B. R. "The Changing Relationship between dominance and social acceptability during group Democratization". *Amer. J. Orthopsychiatry.* 1942, *12*, 529. (It is noted that the children in this study were high-grade mental defectives).

case the children lived in cottages, some of which were run by the children themselves, and some by adults. The form of organisation in the children-directed cottages was recognised as "democratic" inasmuch as they had self-government, while that of the adult-directed cottages was interpreted as "autocratic". It was found that in the "autocratic" cottages the children that showed the most dominant behaviour were those who were the most popular or socially acceptable. This confirmed the general hypothesis that in an autocratic group the relationship between dominative behaviour and popularity would be high. The reason for this relationship being that in an atmosphere or tradition of autocracy the impulse for power is connected with social support. In other words the form of organisation places a premium on the very motive that makes it what it is. The experiment was then made that in one of the adult-directed cottages there was a return to self-government. After four months the relationship between dominance and popularity dropped considerably, and after a further period of increasing democratisation, dropped further still.

A reading of these two studies and similar investigations does not leave one with the strong impression that would otherwise be gathered from a book, say, as Nietzsche's *Thus Spake Zarathustra,* of the inner desire for power. What these studies do bring out is the network of relationships, both between groups and individuals, which is incorporated in the pursuit of dominance. This has the effect of reflecting the emphasis away from the purely individual part of power towards the social aspects.

Power as a Need. An exception to this has been the psychology of Adler,[9] who was one of the first psycho-analysts to bring to the fore the power-striving characteristics of people. The substitution of power for sex as being the chief determinant of man's actions represented the main deviancy of Adler from the doctrines of Freud. Originally Adler formulated his ideas about power in a consideration of "organ inferiority". A person who was born a cripple might tend to compensate for this deficiency by over-developing some other part of his body. A stutterer, by overcoming his default, would go to the other extreme and become a

[9] Adler, A. *The Practice and Theory of Individual Psychology.* Kegan Paul, 1929. For an introduction to Adler's psychology, see Lewis Way: *Alfred Adler: His Psychology.* Pelican Books, 1956.

great orator. Demosthenes is the classical example of this. In his later writings Adler stressed that a feeling of inferiority was universal in man and that a form of domination was a real need in order to compensate for it. This might be done at the expense of somebody else, or it might be achieved by a successful victory over the customary difficulties of life. Alternatively, the striving for superiority might be performed in a fictitious manner, by fantasy and day-dreaming, instead of struggling with reality. This is a theme which in its lighter side has been taken up in such fiction as *Don Quixote* and *The Secret Life of Walter Mitty*. There is no doubt that Adler tended to over emphasise the role of the inferiority-superiority polarity in the life of people, but his insistence on the struggle for power indicates the deeper aspects of this motive.

ACHIEVEMENT

"The achieve of, the mastery of the thing", wrote Gerard Manley Hopkins, a line which epitomises the fact that there is an inherent satisfaction in merely getting something done, whether it is in building a coal bunker, weaving a rug or writing a poem. Such a satisfaction is known to everybody. What is not known to everybody are the individual differences involved in achievement, of the way in which people set themselves ends to be attained. The notion of "levels of aspiration" refers to this fact that people set themselves goals, either consciously or unconsciously, to which they endeavour to reach. These can be either of a major order, such as the acquirement of a professional status, in which case it would be a relatively long-term goal, or of a minor order and a relatively short-term goal such as winning a golf championship. The concept of a level of aspiration can be given very exact experimental expression and can be duplicated in performances in the laboratory with simple tests such as letter-number substitutions or arithmetical problems or solving mazes. A homely example can suffice to exemplify the technical terms used with the notion. A man habitually gets out of bed at nine o'clock which makes him miss his breakfast in order that he gets to work on time. He decides to alter his habit by setting a new level of aspiration of rising at six o'clock. The difference between the level of the last performance and the level of the new goal is called "goal discrepancy". In this example the goal discrepancy is three hours. However he fails to wake up at the time of the new goal, that is six o'clock, but gets up at seven. The difference between the level of the new goal and that of the new performance is called the "attainment discrepancy". In our example this is just one hour. Then comes the reaction to the attainment discrepancy in which there are large individual differences. There are feelings of success or failure, of elatement or disappointment, according to the nature of the individual person. Some people, using our example, will remain satisfied with what they have achieved although it falls short of their previous aspiration. In other words they will set the new hour of waking at seven o'clock in the knowledge that they can achieve this, in which case the fresh attainment discrepancy will be zero. Other people are more persistent and will make repeated attempts to continue with their goal, getting up at six o'clock. Others again, disappointed at their failure, will give up the endeavour altogether and continue rising at nine. Speaking very broadly, the average tendency is to put one's goal just ahead of one's attainment. Also it can be seen that the person who habitually places his goal far higher than he ever achieves lays himself open to all the conditions associated with frustration. However, there are a number of factors related to the level of aspiration which must be taken into account, such as the social background, the standards of the individual's group, and the temperament of a person.[10]

Although the concept of level of aspiration can be given exact quantitative expression with simple laboratory tests, it is possible to adapt it in a qualitative manner. One might apply the idea to people who are continually running into debt for instance. The activity of such people perennially involves the setting of fresh decisions to which they hope to adhere. An examination of their attainment in the light of their new goals can be fruitful. Also it must be remembered that society itself sets levels to which its members react in their individual ways.

SECURITY

There are different modes of security as expressed by the desire of a child for care and affection (a theme which will be discussed in a further section), by the quest for financial safety either in terms of plain cash or in holding down a job, or by the desire for

[10] For a discussion of these factors see Lewin, K. and others "Level of Aspiration", in Hunt, J. M. *Personality and the Behavior Disorders* Vol. 1. Ronald Press, 1944.

"belongingness" either to a group or to some accepted standard of values.

Economic. A feeling of economic insecurity has psychological ramifications far beyond the actual need for £ s. d. and the associated lack of material wants. Loss of the customary financial resources can alter a person's capacity to deal with everyday affairs in an effective manner and can change his position in the family group.[11] Also it has been found that the emotional attitude of children toward their parents in feeling tone, dependency and emotional expression, varied according to the economic level of the family.[12] In this study the attitude of the children of the poorest class towards their parents were the least balanced in terms of the usual standards of mental health.

Group "belongingness". The economic aspect of security is perhaps obvious; there are more explicitly psychological facets which are less apparent. One of these is the security felt in clinging to an accepted body of values or the support from society. There is a certain security in the knowledge that others think alike and will support one's own view. Alternatively to stand alone is a feat which is not easy, requires moral courage, and can be associated with emotional insecurity. The feeling of "belongingness" is a common feature of experience. Without it a person tends to become like the man in the rhyme who complained "I wish that my room had a floor. I don't so much care for a door. But this floating around without touching the ground is getting to be quite a bore!" The emphasis has been put on the perceptual side in this feeling of insecurity.[13] Cartwright suggests that it is determined by two sets of factors. A person has a self-perception of the strength of his own power together with a perception of the support that he thinks he will get, on the one hand, and on the other hand opposing these is the perception of the power from unfriendly sources. These two forces acting as a ratio impinge on a person's feeling of insecurity. It can be seen that as the denominator of the perception of opposition increases, the feeling of

[11] Hoey, J. M. "Social Security". *Amer. J. Orthopsychiatry* 1947, *17*, 426.
[12] Meltzer, H. "Economic Security and Children's Attitudes to Parents". *Amer. J. Orthopsychiatry* 1936, *6*, 590. The point, however, needs further enquiry.
[13] Cartwright, D. "Emotional dimensions of Group Life". in Reymert, M. L. *Feelings and Emotions.* McGraw-Hill, 1950.

security diminishes. The insistence on the perceptual side is important because a feeling of security or insecurity can be at actual variance with the real situation. The feeling is associated with the way in which a person "sees" a situation. There can be the case where a feeling of insecurity is prompted by events that are almost wholly illusional.

MOTIVES IN ADOPTION AND FOSTERING

The need for parenthood and the desire for the company of children are states which are extremely difficult to assess, and about which we have little knowledge. However, the studies[14] that have been made in this field tell us a little about human motives and the subsequent reaction relative to the motive. With adoption a common motive is the condition where no child has been born and the married couple turn to adoption as the only means. This often becomes "the prelude to successful conception of a natural child, whose appearance is greeted with joy, and whose position of ascendancy over the adopted child is all too likely to develop, though perhaps unrecognised by the parents." Another reason for adoption is connected with the death of a child, and the parents want to replace their loss. This can result in disappointment if the new child fails to come up to the expected standards. It has also been noted that parents will adopt children as playmates for their own child, or even to "help someone out" with an illegitimate child.

In fostering, a common motive is what the investigators have called "Declared Altruism". It is disclosed that when some case of child neglect or cruelty is published, there are nearly always a large number of people who volunteer to foster the child. This has repercussions in that pity is a motive that makes for difficulties. To quote the authors at this point: "It is said that 'pity is akin to love', but it is also akin to cruelty. Thus many people with unconscious sadistic tendencies of their own are so emotionally pitiful of the victims of similar tendencies in others that they seek to counteract their own guilt by offering to foster the ill-treated

[14] The material for these paragraphs has been taken from three reports by the Southampton Discussion Group of social workers. "Motives in Adoption". *Social Work* 1952, *9*, 669 and 689, and "Motives in Fostering" *Social Work* 1952, *9*, 733. The United Nations publication *Study on Adoption of Children* 1953 has also been consulted. The necessity remains, however, for a large-scale reliable investigation of motives in adoption and fostering.

child. Unfortunately the child when boarded out may all too soon display the characteristics that gave rise to the cruelty in the first place and because pity may be the obverse side of sadism the last condition will be as bad as the first."

Another motive in fostering is the feeling of loneliness in the parent. This seldom has beneficial consequences and places a strain on the child. Yet another reason for fostering (and adoption also) which often results in failure is the desire to have a child in order to avoid a breakdown of the marriage.

The above list only represents a bare classification that has been found in a relatively small number of prospective parents. A proper evaluation of the motives in this sphere of human relationships is contingent on a great deal of further evidence.

VALUES

Although the subject of values pertains strictly to systems of philosophy, the psychological approach consists in the enquiry of the type of preferences which people hold. Everybody has some kind of values, whether these are gained from an understanding of personal experience or from an uncritical acceptance of the principles that have been laid down in childhood.

The psychological study of values has been made both from a consideration of personality types, and from the wider viewpoint of the prevailing standards in the culture and sub-cultures. We will discuss both of these in turn.

TYPES OF MEN

A notable example of the first approach was the work of Spranger[15] who attempted to classify men by the types of values to which they adhered. He listed six types: the theoretical, the economic, the æsthetic, the social, the political, and the religious man.

Theoretical Type. By this type, Spranger denotes a man whose dominant interest is the discovery of truth, whose attitude is mainly intellectual, pre-eminently an observer and man of reason. The picture is that of an intellectual, scientist or philosopher, a person whose interests are empirical, critical and rational. A good

[15] Spranger, E. *Types of Men.* 1928 trans.

22

self-evaluative example of this kind of person is given by Einstein, who in some autobiographical notes[16] (which he called an obituary and which contained little to no facts about his personal life) wrote: " 'Is this supposed to be an obituary?' the astonished reader will likely ask. I would like to reply: essentially yes. For the essential in the being of a man of my type lies precisely in *what* he thinks and *how* he thinks, not in what he does or suffers."

Economic Type. Spranger's second type, the economic man, is a person whose interests are essentially practical. The applied scientist, the business man, and the person who has an impatience with affairs of "mere theory", all fit into this type. In a condensed version of the Spranger list, Vernon and Allport[17] describe this type as frequently coming into conflict with other values: "The economic man wants education to be practical, and regards unapplied knowledge as waste. . . . The value of utility likewise conflicts with the asthetic value, excepting when art serves commercial ends. Without feeling inappropriateness in his act, the economic man may denude a beautiful hillside or befoul a river with industrial refuse. In his personal life he is likely to confuse luxury with beauty. In his relations with people he is more likely to be interested in surpassing them in wealth than in dominating them (political attitude) or in serving them (social attitude)."

Æsthetic Type. The third type is the æsthetic. His experiences are judged from the point of view of grace, symmetry, or fitness. His chief interest is in the artistic episodes of life, although he need not be a creative artist. An interest in people (though not necessarily in their welfare), a love of pomp, a passion for individualism are further marks of the æsthetic man. "Art for Art's sake" is, perhaps, the credo of this type of man.

Social Type. The dominant motive of the social man, the fourth type, is a love of people, a tendency towards altruism and philanthropy. He takes other people as ends in themselves and is therefore kind, sympathetic and unselfish.

[16] Einstein, A. Autobiographical Notes. In Schilpp: *Albert Einstein: Philosopher Scientist.* Tudor Publishing Co. 1951.

[17] Vernon, P. E. and Allport, G. W. A test for Personal Values *J. Abn. Soc. Psychol.* 1931, *26*, 231.

Political Type. In contrast to the social man who regards other people as ends, the fifth type, the political man, accepts them as means. This type is interested in power, though he may not be a politician. Indeed he might very well be a priest (a "grey eminence") or a scholar (like Dr. Faustus). The emphasis is on power and influence, a mastery over people and affairs.

Religious Type. The sixth and final type is the religious man, the mystic, a man who finds his aim and end in life in religious experience.

It is to be noted that Spranger's ideal types are characterised by the mental structure and inner purpose of the person idealised, and not necessarily by what they have done, by their achievements. There is no doubt that other types might have been envisaged, and that many people could be categorised as belonging to two or more of the types, or a mixture of all of them. But the classification has proved to be useful in psychology. Allport and Vernon[18] have devised a questionnaire using Spranger's ideal types as its basis, in order to measure the prominence of fundamental motives and evaluative attitudes. Following this initial study there have been numerous other investigations, using the same method of approach.

Values and Interests. Occupational interest has been found to bear on the original value-types of Spranger as used on the Allport-Vernon questionnaire. A number of studies have been made with the idea of correlating the occupation with the value-type, and it has been found generally that certain classes of occupations have a predominant attached value. Thus researches have shown that economic values were shared by the interests of office clerks, lawyers and public accountants; theoretical values were linked with schoolteachers, engineers, and people having the same interests as physicians; people with interests similar to nurses had high social and low æsthetic values. Eysenck[19], in citing these and other studies, has summed up the relationship between values and interests as follows: "The evidence is fairly conclusive that values as measured by the Allport-Vernon Scale are closely related to interest patterns . . . people's values, as measured by

[18] *op. cit.*
[19] Eysenck, H. J. *The Psychology of Politics.* Routledge and Kegan Paul 1954.

the Allport-Vernon Scale, are structured in a manner which is very similar to that indicated by attitude studies; and that vocational interests also agree to a remarkable extent with this pattern." Social values (taking the term more than the connotation given to it by Spranger) have been found to ramify into selection of groups of friends, occupations and interests. It is not surprising that they have a wide generality. The majority of people are not in the position of the Miller of Dee; everyone cares for someone (if not everyone) or something, so that value systems inevitably come into play, in one's work, in one's leisure activity, whenever there is an inter-relationship of people.

CULTURAL DIVERSITY

For those who wish to study the role of value systems in human affairs, the facts culled from cultures other than one's own encourages a wider outlook. No less for the social worker than the psychologist, sociologist or anthropologist, this is a focal matter. Value judgements inevitably creep in when dealing with matters of pure fact, and although in theory a worker is presumed not to allow his or her judgement to be influenced by group or class factors, there always exists an implicit framework of categories against which judgements or assessments are made. Therefore to be reminded that people exist who hold ideas remarkably different from our own is often salutary.

Co-operative versus Competitive Values. Many examples of differing value systems throughout the world could be cited; one set of contrasting values can be given with respect to the economic and social side of the community. This is the case where the society places importance to co-operation on the one hand and competition on the other.[20] The Zuni Indians in the south-west of the United States, for example, are characterised by a dislike of individual competitive behaviour. Property is communal, and individual success is regarded as shameful. In fact a person who displays a large amount of initiative is considered abnormal and comes under the suspicion of witchcraft. In contrast, the Kwakiutl Indians of the north-west United States and western Canada have

---

[20] see Newcomb, T. M. *Social Psychology*. Tavistock Pubns. 1950. Taken in turn from Mead, M. *Co-operation and Competition among Primitive Peoples.* 1937. See also Benedict, R. *Patterns of Culture*. G. Routledge 1934.

a very powerful competitive society. Here the emphasis is on prestige; achievement in a personal sense determines the individual's position in society. A member of these Indians will go to any length to instal himself high in prestige value in relation to his fellows. While the conduct of the individual Zuni is marked by convention and moderation, the Kwakiutl Indian oscillates from the opposite poles of victory over others and shame when defeated by others. In these two contrasting societies can be seen the relationship of conduct to the values of society; what is proper and correct for one culture is not for another.

DIVERSITY IN SUB-CULTURES

It has been shown that this last statement holds true even for societies within any one culture. What is deprecated by people in one sub-culture is more positively received in another. To understand people's conduct it is often necessary to regard it in the light of the values of the society from which they come.

Values and Delinquency. Mays[21] in his study of juvenile delinquency in certain areas within Liverpool, was struck by the fact that "Delinquency has become almost a social tradition and it is only a very few youngsters who are able to grow up in these areas without at some time or other committing illegal acts." A higher proportion of boys in these areas underwent a delinquent phase than in the rest of the city. The author goes on to argue that "delinquency is not so much a symptom of maladjustment as of adjustment to a sub-culture in conflict with the culture of the city as a whole. The need for the individual to conform to the standards and conventions of the group is very marked and where the activities of the juvenile group have delinquent tendencies it is inevitable that the individual should exhibit the same symptoms." The important point to be noted from this study is that anti-social activities such as shoplifting do not carry with it the over-tones of misdemeanour which the law and other people give it. As one boy said "Shoplifting is regarded more as a sport and an adventure than as crime." Nevertheless there existed in the boys of these areas a scale of values. Thus one boy said that "he wouldn't think twice about stealing from large stores because

[21] Mays, J. B. *Growing up in the City.* University Press of Liverpool 1954.

they rob you with their fantastic prices", but it was thought definitely wrong to steal from friends and associates.

A similar finding of differing standards held within one area was noted by investigators of juvenile delinquency in a working class town in the Midlands.[22] Within working class areas in this town there were two extreme values maintained, in two streets within two minutes' walk of each other, "Dyke Street" and "Gladstone Road". In other words, as the report said "Dyke Street and Gladstone Road, in fact, constitute two well-defined sub-cultures, exhibiting in many directions contrasting ways of life." The attitude towards family life and responsibilities, towards the law, and towards sexual behaviour is remarkably different, in each of these streets. This study represents yet another vivid example of the diversity of values that can be held even within a limited geographical area.

Peer Group Values. The individual is influenced in the selection of his values by the over-all tradition of the culture and sub-culture, as we have seen. Within these the impact of family customs, school teaching and the values of groups composed of individuals of the same age and status (peer groups), all have their effect. In adolescence the functions of peer groups, which can take the form of cliques or sets or even gangs, are very important for the formation of values. They can either support adult and family values or be at variance with them. In either direction they are an important agency of socialisation.

It might be thought that the selection of a peer group may depend upon the values of the family in the first place. A study[23] made with boys from Working Class and Middle Class families indicated that this was not so. In response to a questionnaire asking for desirable qualities in friends, the results did show that there was a definite relationship between the class values of the family and that of the *hypothetical* choice of a friend. There was a difference in the choice of qualities which were regarded as desirable in friends between Middle Class and Working Class

---

[22] University of Nottingham: *The Social Background of Delinquency* 1954. Arthur Morrison's Novel *A Child of the Jago*. Penguin Books 1946, first published in 1896, portraying a section of Shoreditch, gives a good picture of "street-values".

[23] Oppenheim, A. N. "Social Status and Clique Formation among Grammar School Boys". *Brit. J. Sociol.* 1955, 6, 228.

boys. But although this was a *considered* judgement, *actual* friend-ship groupings were found *not* to be influenced by the family values. There is an important element in this discrepancy, for it would suggest that in young people class values are not so en-crusted in the personality as to make responses to the value systems of other people a difficult task, and that *ascribed* values of social class may be no more than lip-service to the implicit assumptions of family background.

FRUSTRATION AND CONFLICT

Common experience tells us that we seldom have wishes or impulses without some obstruction to their attainment. Also life is rarely so simple that we do not have contradictory impulses, so that the choice between two motives becomes a matter of opposition. These two conditions we call frustration and conflict respectively. We will discuss each in turn in this section, but there is an important subject, namely the reaction to frustration and conflict, which will be discussed in Chapter VI in the section entitled "Psycho-Analytic Aspects".

FRUSTRATION

The sources of frustration may be due either to obstacles in the environment which act as a barrier to the satisfaction of an im-pulse, or to personal defects which act as internal barriers.

Environmental Obstacles. This source of frustration may occur either because a desired object is lacking, or that a desired object is unable to be gained. A child, for example, may be frustrated in its desire for an ice-cream either because there are no ice-creams in the vicinity or because its parents disallow the buying of one. The first kind of obstacle is simply physical, the second is social. A famine or drought are obvious examples of physical obstruc-tions leading to the frustration of physiological needs; the law is a prime example of a social obstruction. Often the two may act in conjunction as in the case of rationing when a commodity is scarce.

Personal Defects. Frustration may occur because of a barrier within the individual himself. This may be either grossly physical, as in

28

the case of a cripple wishing to perform actions which are impossible for him (we will take up this aspect more in the next section), or it may be more psychological. An abnormally shy person may suffer agonies in his desire to communicate by being continually thwarted owing to his feelings of making a fool of himself. There is also the situation when a person is committed to a line of action for which he is not suited. A young man who is persuaded to enter the medical profession merely on the strength of family pressure, because the tradition of the family has been that of becoming doctors, may suffer frustration on account of his failure to make the grade due either to a lack of genuine interest or a personal intellectual inadequacy. In fact many frustrations may occur in the choice of occupations unsuitable to a person's temperament or intelligence.

Frustration and Aggression. The assumption has been made[24] that aggression is the result of frustration. By this is meant that interference to the satisfaction of reaching a goal results in a pent-up tension which is then released in a negative way. A simple example is illustrated by people who are unrequited in love and who then "take it out" on others around them. A more elaborate example is that given by Dollard when he suggests that people who are deprived of their liberty and suffer excessive restrictions, as under a totalitarian regime, tend to be abnormally aggressive. Although it is the State which enforces the frustration, aggression cannot be directed against it, owing to internal suppression, so the aggression is channelled to a socially permitted target, such as the Jews or capitalists.

Although there is a certain amount of evidence in favour of this assumption, it is by no means certain that every type of aggression is caused by frustration, nor that frustration always leads to aggression. Frustration results in a number of reactions, one of which *may* be aggression. As we shall see in the next section there are other possibilities. Moreover it should be made clear that what amounts to a frustration may differ from individual to individual, not only in what each regards as a frustration but also as to the amount of similar obstructions each has had in the past. One

[24] First by Freud who later changed his opinion, but more fully by Dollard, J. and others. *Frustration and Aggression.* Kegan Paul 1939. The hypothesis was modified by Miller, N. E. "The Frustration Aggression Hypothesis". *Psychol. Review* 1941, *48*, 337.

common obstruction may be the first of its kind to one person, to another it may be the "last straw". Also the situation is important. As Himmelweit[25] emphasises, "Situational factors play a role in determining the intensity of a frustration experience. An experience, shared with another person, is usually felt to be less frustrating. Not only the interpersonal relationship of co-sufferers but also that between the subject and the person responsible for the frustration, is important. A prohibition made by a teacher, invested with authority, will be felt by the child quite differently from the same prohibition made by the mother." In short there are a number of conditions which affect the determination of frustration and which similarly influence its connection with aggression.

CONFLICT OF MOTIVES

Another source of frustration is the conflict of motives within an individual. Conflicting motives may be of different types and we shall first therefore have to provide a classification. There are a number of ways of doing this, but we shall quote Newcomb's[26] analysis, as this classification fits in with what has already been discussed about frustration.

Classification. Newcomb establishes four types of conflict according as to whether they are goal-oriented or threat-oriented. The first is what he labels "Appeal-appeal". Here there are two alternative goals of equal desirability. The story of Buridan's Ass who could not choose between two bundles of hay and starved as a result is a good example of this type. It is sometimes seen in a child who is faced with the delicious choice of an ice-cream or a lollipop; he cannot make up his mind and decides on both—a selection which is seldom countenanced by the parent! The second type, "Threat-threat", is, as Newcomb says, characterised by finding oneself between the devil and the deep blue sea. Hamlet's dilemma—to be or not to be—is the classical instance.

The third type is "Appeal with threat". A positive line of

[25] Himmelweit, H. T. "Frustration and Aggression". In Pear, T. H. *Psychological Factors of Peace and War*. Hutchinson 1950.

[26] Newcomb, T. M. *Social Psychology*. Tavistock 1950. Newcomb's classification is very similar to that first made by Kurt Lewin: *A Dynamic theory of Personality*. McGraw-Hill 1935. Lewin's basic types were called "approach-approach conflict, avoidance-avoidance conflict, and approach-avoidance conflict."

action has its negative aspect. The forbidden fruit has its attractions. The goal which has its satisfactions cannot be gained except with the acceptance of consequences which are undesirable. Any course of action which entails a certain amount of pain is tabled under this category; this may be in a lesser or greater degree. Accepting the fact that one must visit the dentist to relieve a painful tooth represents a relatively small conflict; the decision, by someone in authority, to send men to a dangerous situation, may well prove a relatively big conflict. The fourth type, "Multiple Appeals with threats", is an elaboration of the third type but complicated by the fact that there are many alternatives. Newcomb comments that "This type of conflict, like the others, results not so much from the actual possibilities which confront a person as from the ways in which he perceives the possibilities. Some individuals, faced with alternatives each of which involves both threat and appeal, characteristically minimize the risks. Others brood over them and scarcely dwell at all upon the possibilities of gain. For the latter kind of person, this fourth type of conflict becomes in fact the second type, that of threat vs. threat."

Conflict between values. As we have seen a person may gain his values from various sources. The question now is formed; what happens when these are conflicting? A typical instance might be the values that have been inculcated in the family conflicting with those demanded by society. Very often these are in harmony, but one can imagine the situation of an adolescent whose family background has been that of varying forms of criminality faced with the desire to conform to the conventional values of society. Conflicts between values owing to the different sub-cultures in society can be numerous. Different racial, national and religious backgrounds provide sets of values that may be at complete variance with the standards of society. Minority groups can be at continual strife with the rest of the community with which they share the same environment. Value conflicts of this nature can be resolved for the individual by the feeling of security within the family; conversely if there is a feeling of insecurity in the family then the conflict of values may be increased.

It has been pointed out[27] how contradictory values attached to

[27] By Merton, R. K. *Social Theory and Social Structure* 1949. Quoted by Broom, L. and Selznick, P. *Sociology*. Row, Peterson and Co. 1956.

ends and means can lead to criminalistic actions. Thus in contemporary American culture there is a high premium put on the accumulation of wealth, and success is highly valued; at the same time the values attached to the *legal* means of achieving these ends make achievement of them impossible for many members of the lower classes. Therefore *illegal* means are resorted to. Commenting on this in their textbook of Sociology, Broom and Selznick present the following sequence: "(1) Certain groups are in poverty; they are unable to attain many of the material goods which their culture stresses as important. (2) These groups, then, lose respect for and loyalty to the values which, if maintained, deny 'success' to them. (3) Since success is measured in terms of property, the loss of respect for society's values is a dissociation from or lack of respect for the 'property rights' of the culture. (4) Disrespect for property rights, in turn, results in a high incidence of crimes against property."

Conflict between roles. We shall discuss the concept of "role" in the Chapter on Personality; for the present we shall define it as the pattern of behaviour that a person is expected to carry out as a result of occupying a position in society. The role of a policeman, for example, is to enforce the laws of society. Now conflict between roles comes about because it can happen that a person may occupy two or even more positions at the same time, and the roles attached to these positions are incompatible. A classic historical example of a role conflict was that of Sir Thomas More, the author of *Utopia*, who as Lord Chancellor was called upon to condone the divorce of Henry VIII and subsequent marriage to Anne Boleyn, but who as devout churchman could not allow this.

In this case the conflict was resolved by resignation from the political office. Another type of role conflict can be seen in industry, where a foreman is often in the unenviable position of carrying out the wishes of his employers against the desires of his fellow workers. In these and similar situations, a conflict does not properly develop unless there is some doubt in a person's mind as to which way he should turn. It might be said of Sir Thomas More that there was very little actual conflict here because the dictates of his conscience came clearly first. Where there is a clear hierarchy of roles the conflict between them is not likely to develop to a degree which is alarming. It is the case where there is genuine ambiguity that provides serious opposition.

CONFLICT IN THE FAMILY

Conflict within the family can take place (1) Between parents and children (2) Between the children themselves (3) Between the spouses, that is marital conflict.

In one sense the whole of upbringing is a series of conflicts between the child and its parents. These, however, are relatively minor upsets which are part and parcel of any family. Serious conflicts arise when the child is rejected by one or both of its parents. There can be several varieties of rejection.[28] The parents may be openly antagonistic to the child: the parents may be antagonistic, but their antagonism is directed not so much to the child itself as to its behaviour: one parent may overtly reject the child while the other parent spoils him: a parent may adopt a vacillating attitude, ranging from over-indulgence at one time to sharp criticism at another: finally the child may simply suffer from lack of affection. In all these cases frustration and conflict can develop, and difficulties of behaviour can further develop according to the attitudes of the parents. If a generalisation can be made from the observational studies made on the attitude of parents towards their children, it is that not only does a child require love and affection for its normal development, but that ambiguity regarding its position in the family should not be allowed to develop.

Another type of conflict between parents and children arises at a later stage of development of the latter when the values of the family are rejected in favour of another group. This happens very often in adolescence, and is perhaps a phenomenon common enough not to warrant further discussion. It is sufficient to point out that the conflict in this case comes from an allegiance to the values of one group while still having to conform to the set of values of another (family) group.

Sibling Rivalry. Psycho-analytic thought assumes that there is a competition between siblings for the love of the desired parent.

[28] Taken from Witmer, H. L. "Parental behavior as an index to the probable outcome of treatment in a Child Guidance Clinic". *Amer. J. Orthopsychiatry* 1933, *3*, 431.

In the ordinary way it is very difficult to assess children's intentions through their own formulations. Jealousy of the new baby is a commonly observed phenomenon. What we wish to know is something further than this. Levy[29] surmounted the difficulty of communication with children in matters like this by providing the children with dolls, which symbolised children. The type of procedure he used is illustrated by the example of a boy watching dolls representing a baby at its mother's breast and an older child as himself. The boy is asked "And then the brother sees the new baby at the mother's breast. He never saw him before. What does he do?" Responses to this question vary remarkably. There is sometimes enacted the "complete primitive performance" as Levy puts it, in which the doll is attacked by the child and destroyed. He noticed that often there is a tendency to destroy but the child is kept back by inhibitions. Then too there is another type of response. The doll representing the subject himself is slapped. Asked why, the answer comes, "because she (the subject this time is a girl) was bad. She wanted to hit the baby".

There are many children who of course are the reverse of this and tend to behave towards the new baby and other siblings quite differently. All that we wish to outline here is that sibling rivalry is just as important a source of conflict within the family as that between parents and children.

Marital Conflict. Conflict between the partners of a marriage contract has so long been the butt of books, plays, cartoons and the music hall, that it almost seems a further parody to attempt to posit psychological explanations. Also it is clear that we are presented with difficulties of a methodological nature. The material presented in the present section has been gained at very different investigatory levels. A question like marital conflict is obviously not open to experimental investigation in the laboratory. What is possible is to make assumptions from a study of many different cases seen in a clinic. Theoretical explanations can then be made with respect to them but obviously they are not simple to verify. Notwithstanding these difficulties attempts have been made to generalise from observations of a number of cases, and verification

[29] Levy, D. M. "Studies in Sibling Rivalry". *Res. Monog. Amer. Orthopsych. Assoc.* 1937 No. 2. "The Hostile Act" in Newcomb, T. M. and Hartley, E. L. *Readings in Social Psychology.* Holt 1947.

has been made through the application of advice or some mild therapeutic measure. For instance Dicks[30] has put forward the generalisation that "marital disharmony is frequently the expression of dominance-submission conflicts rooted in discrepancy between role and unconscious needs". There is the whole range of personal desires and needs of the marital partner; at the same time there is the particular role of husband or wife which has to be played. Disharmony becomes, then, a matter of discrepancy between the husband or wife as a *person* and *as* husband or wife. Dicks pursues this theme to maintain that the conflict is contained in the need for dominance or passivity with respect to the role. This is internal initially but can become externalised in the marital relation. To quote him fully "We may see in the struggle for ascendancy among a married couple the projection of a bad object (such as a frustrating parent) or denials in one or both of them of their own deeper needs by a process of over-compensation. The partner may be attacked as if he or she were a frustrator in order to justify the subject's own aggressive feelings towards the object, and to ward off guilt at the failure in role fulfillment."

That the factor of passivity is analogous to over-dependence is remarked upon by Hollis[31] in her study of the role of women in marital conflict. She notes that too close parental ties are one of the personality factors involved in marital conflict. A woman who is excessively dependent has the inability to be generous in love, has the drawback of having the need to be given affection before she can offer it, has an inability to forgive and on the other hand clings to "the empty shell of a marriage" because of the fear for the unknown. Also pertinent is the transference of a dependence upon parents to that of the husband, who, as Hollis points out, is seldom emotionally strong enough to take this burden.

These studies do underline the viewpoint that although economic difficulties, cultural differences and the intervention of parents and friends undoubtedly have influence on the relation between the spouses, the prime factor is that of personality difficulties, no less here than in other types of family conflict.

[30] Dicks, H. V. "Clinical studies in marriage and the family: a symposium on methods: I. Experiences with marital tension seen in the Psychological Clinic". *Brit. J. Med. Psych.* 1953, *26*, 181. Not all cases of marital tension are of the dominance-submission type it should be stressed.

[31] Hollis, F. *Women in Marital Conflict: A Casework Study.* 1949. Family Service Association of America.

This entire matter has lately been raised in a report by a group of caseworkers[32] and further elaboration seems unnecessary in the light of this. It does seem necessary to emphasise one aspect which this group has noticed, namely the fact that many marital relationships have been made on the level of fantasy. As they put it "Development to a mature level of relationship within the marriage may be especially difficult if the choice has been made in phantasy terms on both sides, and the persistence of deep-seated anxieties or guilt compels the partners to maintain their unconscious 'collusion' to keep the relationship in these terms." The conflict between the levels of irreality or fantasy and that of brute empirical facts of daily living results in a lack of harmony that reflects itself in many fields. In marriage it would seem to be particularly relevant, especially in those cases where the husband or wife have been unconsciously biased by assimilating the ideal values in books and films. Hollywood and some weekly magazines are not necessarily the best of standards upon which to base selection of marital partners or to assess the requirements in a husband or wife. Whether it is bad or good, the fact remains that this undoubtedly occurs in some cases, and is a point which must not be overlooked in marital problems.

PRIVATION

Having considered some of the goals to which people are orientated and some of the means they take to reach them, we now turn to the position when these goals are persistently withdrawn from a person's attainment and when basic human needs are not satisfied. The causes of deprivation may range from a lack of a part of the body to the loss of a parent, and from a deficiency in intake of food to loss of liberty. The effects of privation may differ considerably. Some people are all the better for having had a bad time; with others it leaves a permanent trace. This, of course, depends upon the degree of hardship involved, and it may be that there is a point beyond which the human organism cannot bear, although reports of people tortured indicate how much a person can actually bear, a degree which is often surprising.

[32] Bannister, K. and others. Family Discussion Bureau. *Social Casework in Marital Problems*. Tavistock Publications 1955.

General Effects of Privation. Sherif[33] has outlined the effects of some forms of deprivation. The particular goal of which the person is deprived tends to colour his perceptions, memories, imagination and conduct (to the extent that is possible); he may resort to substitute activity and to fantasy; and finally if the deprivation continues beyond certain limits, to a breakdown of the usually accepted social values. Bettleheim, who himself had spent some years in the concentration camps of Nazi Germany and yet somehow managed to make systematic observations, has vividly described such a breakdown. Not only was there a regression to infantile behaviour and a tendency towards identification with the torturers among the older prisoners, but there was a re-valuation of experience in terms of earlier, less mature, behaviour. "Prisoners seemed, for instance, particularly sensitive to punishments similar to those which a parent might inflict on his child. To punish a child was within their 'normal' frame of reference, but that they should become the object of the punishment destroyed their adult frame of reference. So they reacted to it not in an adult, but in a childish way—with embarrassment and shame, with violent, impotent and unmanageable emotions directed, not against the system, but against the person inflicting the punishment." This is a very extreme case and the instances which will be quoted below do not reach this degree of intensity. Extreme examples do help, however, to bring out the salient features of a principle which less marked instances fail to.

Another example of the effects of privation was provided by an experimental "famine" carried out in the Laboratory of Physiological Hygiene, University of Minnesota, by a number of investigators.[34] Volunteers were systematically starved for a period of six months, to the extent of losing twenty-five per cent of their original weight. The physical results need not concern us. Some of the psychological results indicated an increase of irritability and moroseness. Complaints were frequent, one of the more interesting ones being the sensation of feeling "old". There was a breakdown of moral values among some of the men, there was stealing of food and breaking of the rules of voluntary diet. Individuals became more remote from one another and developed a dislike for

[33] Sherif, M. *An Outline of Social Psychology.* Harper 1948. Bettleheim, B. "Individual and Mass Behaviour in extreme situations". *J. Abn. Soc. Psychol.* 1943, *38*, 417.
[34] Keys, A. and others. *Experimental Starvation in Man* 1945. quoted by Sherif. *op. cit.*

strangers. As the report put it: "Although fasting is said at times to quicken one spiritually, none of the men reported significant progress in their religious lives. Most of them felt that the semi-starvation had coarsened rather than refined them, and they marvelled at how thin their moral and social veneers seemed to be."

THE HANDICAPPED CHILD

A quite different form of privation, and one which represents a continual problem to the social services is that of the handicapped child. We shall interpret the term "handicapped" in a broad way, including under its rubric severe cases such as paralyses and blindness to the more minor defects. We shall consider the privation of these children from the point of view of the attitude of others towards them, and the connection of this with their handicap.

Social Perception. At the outset it should be noticed with Barker[35] that a person who is generally seen by his associates as disabled is thus socially handicapped. In fact the single indicator of physical disability is defined as follows: "A physically disabled person is one who is *generally perceived* in his cultural group to have a physique that prevents him from participating in *important* activities on terms of *equality* with normal individuals of his own age." This statement throws the focus on social perception, a fact which is important when it comes to considering interpersonal relationships. Social ostracisation may widen the gap that would exist normally between a handicapped child and those about him. Alternatively, it can be ameliorated by social acceptance. Maberly[36] in a discussion of this theme in relation to delinquency, points out that unless there are specific steps taken to assist the handicapped child to overcome the difficulties of inferiority and inadequacy, there is likely to be a distortion of normal development inasmuch that a failure to make personal relationships results in a liability to show anti-social behaviour. Satisfaction of his own needs are gained at the expense of others, to whom there are no feelings of affection or loyalty.

[35] Barker, L. S. and others. "The Frequency of Physical Disability in Children". *Child Development* 1952, *23*, 215.
[36] Maberly, A. "Delinquency in handicapped children". *Brit. J. Delinquency* 1950, *1*, 125.

Parental Attitude. Prior to social acceptance, however, there is the over-riding factor of parental attitude. This seems to be the conclusion to which most studies in this field arrive. Carter and Chess[37] for example in their study of organically ill children who showed behaviour disturbances, stated that the most prominent factor determining whether anxiety developed into an important element was in fact that of the parental attitude. Over-protection in the more dominating parent—usually the mother—was connected with difficulty of relationship of the child with his peers. It was noteworthy that the authors found no predictable relationship between the amount of parental anxiety and the handicap *per se*, nor of anything to do with the handicap as such. Anxiety in the parents seemed more related to their own particular emotional needs and their own fundamental attitudes towards the child.

Rejection of the child may vary in kind. For example, Westlund and Palumbo[38] noted that in a group of cases of infantile paralyses, there were two types of rejection. In the first there was a conscious and overt rejection, with frequent criticism of the child and his behaviour. The second type of rejection is more serious because it is more subtle. The rejection is not at all conscious. It includes those cases where the child, because of his deficiency, is unable to reach the ideals intended for him by the parent, and thus disappoints the parent. A father who wanted his son to be a boxer developed a dislike for the child when he became disabled. Also stressed by these authors is the child's position in the family, what he has meant to the parents and how they have felt towards him.

Rehabilitation. Rehabilitation of handicapped children rests not only on medical methods but also the psychological support of those caring for and treating them. McBroom and Froelich[39] in discussing cases of rheumatic fever with some degree of heart damage have remarked that the most responsive children to adjustment to the new convalescent centre conditions were those who had had opportunities for emotional security and growth with their own parents. This report lays emphasis on the need for

[37] Carter, V. and Chess, S. "Factors influencing the adaptation of organically handicapped children". *Amer. J. Orthopsychiatry.* 1951, *21*, 827.

[38] Westlund, N. and Palumbo, A. Z. "Parental rejection of crippled children". *Amer. J. Orthopsychiatry.* 1946, *16*, 271.

[39] McBroom, E. and Froelich, U. "Interpretation of physical disability to children". *Social Casework* 1949, *30*, 154.

sensitivity and sincerity on the part of the adult, and cites an interesting example when this is not done. "The extent to which these children have been confused by adult temporizing or carelessness in the course of their illness is suggested by the following conversation recorded by a housemother who observed a group of 8- and 9-year-old girls playing 'doctor-and-hospital' with their dolls. All these children had had long periods of hospitalisation and sustained moderate to severe heart damage:

Nancy (*speaking to her doll with affected sweetness*): Now you'll be taken to the hospital, honey. It's just lovely at the hospital.

(*Cynical, derisive laughter from the other three girls*).

Mollie: Does your baby know how sick she is?

Nancy: Of course not. We never tell her that.

Grace: It doesn't matter what we say in front of these babies. Babies don't understand."

As against this there is the positive side of the picture presented by Turner[40] of a Cripples Help Society in the North, which deals with the case of a seven-year-old boy with a severe spinal condition. Here was a child, who through the care and persistence of a teacher, changed from a neglected child with no formal education to a boy who took an interest in nature study and modelling, and almost reached the standard of education expected of his age. And this was done in fifteen months. This interest in the boy not only had an effect on his general appearance and physical condition, but also brought about a change in the mother's attitude. She changed from a "tired apathy" about the child to take a new interest in the boy and also in the appearance of the home. In short over and above actual physical disabilities, there stands the psychological attitude of the disabled child on the one hand, and the disposition of the parents and society as a whole on the other. Whatever may be the position as regards the actual physical nature of the case, the self perception of the child and the perception of others close to him, concerning him, are very influential factors.

ECONOMIC

The psychological effects of unemployment have been subjected to an exhaustive analysis by Eisenberg and Lazarsfeld,[41]

[40] Turner, R. "The Needs of the severely handicapped child". *Social Welfare* 1947, 6, 264.

[41] Eisenberg, P. and Lazarsfeld, P. F. "The Psychological effects of Unemployment". *Psychol. Bulletin* 1938, *35*, 358.

who subdivided the effects into four categories, namely the effects of unemployment on personality, socio-political attitudes affected by unemployment, differing attitudes produced by unemployment and related factors, and the effect of unemployment on children and youth. We need not go into all these; we will note that the main conclusion appears to be that unemployment makes people more emotionally unstable, in comparison to the time when they were not unemployed, and that there is a lowering of morale. One interesting point which the authors note from a study by Rund-quist and Sletto belies the common belief that unemployed men are characterised by feelings of inferiority. This idea should be qualified by the fact that the man out of work has inferiority feelings only when he is aware that unemployment has been selective, and that his own personal deficiencies stand in the way of his getting a job. However, as the writers state, the point needs further research. It is plain that there is a lowering of prestige in situations like this—this is well brought out in Walter Greenwood's novel *Love on the Dole*, where the breadwinner of the family is the daughter, during the unemployment of the father. Psychological effects of poverty and unemployment are perhaps better suited for treatment by novels and plays rather than the systematic study of the social psychologist, inasmuch that the emotional element which is so strong in these cases is put over in a clearer way.

Homelessness and Displacement. What amounts to another form of economic privation is that expressed by homelessness and displacement. It is not only the Englishman whose home is his castle, nor is it necessarily the aged who cling on desperately to their familiar surroundings. In a sense everybody has this feeling of "belongingness" and a rupture of it disturbs the balance of normal life. Unfortunately there are not many studies on this subject that would indicate general principles. The clinging to the old ways of behaviour is seen in a study of displaced persons in Europe by Rimmer,[42] who noticed that there was a clinging to group values and a reverence for old traditions. This is what would have been easily predicted from a knowledge of other areas of social psychology and endorses the fact that there is a very great

[42] Rimmer, J. E. "The meaning of homelessness as seen in a community of displaced persons". *Brit. J. Psychiatric Social Work* 1948 August. No. 2, p. 80.

need to feel at one with society. When a person's usual society is suddenly uprooted, all the customary values and habits of thought and behaviour are uprooted with it. His world collapses about him and it is not surprising that there should be a renewed valuation of the world that he once knew, and a clinging to old ways of acting. Displaced persons present a particular problem to social workers, and although it may not be such a contemporary problem as it undoubtedly was in the years following the recent world war, it is still interesting from a psychological point of view. Berl[43] has made several interesting points about such people from the standpoint of casework. He remarks on the fact that the displaced person client is a cultural stranger and that this sometimes has the result of reacting to the group he belongs to, and as he puts it "it is a cliche reaction", which contains an unconscious cultural bias. From the client's side there is a quandary inasmuch as he is not certain what are the new social and cultural norms and biases. "His experience of cultural bias in his new reality is sharpened because as an immigrant he is a member of a 'weak' social group. A weak group is apt to draw upon itself the aggressive impulses in a community which are held in social control otherwise." Berl continues to stress the peculiar psychological fact that the social worker's reaction to the client is tinged with a feeling of guilt engendered by moral responsibility to the client's group. "The client comes to us for help in separating from his group and the past it represents. However, the worker may not be able to separate himself from this past because of the unresolved moral issue it respresents for him. This may mean that our giving service may become a way of meeting our own need instead of the client's. It also means difficulty in understanding the client's use of his past in his relationship to the worker." Berl is considering mainly the displaced person who has suffered in concentration camps; his observations, however, can be generalised to include less severe forms of displacement.

It can be seen that deprivation of economic needs, whether these be cash or homes has a far reaching effect not only on the person who lacks them himself but also on other people with whom he comes in contact. Deficiencies of this nature leave a mark which is recognised by other people and influences their reactions.

[43] Berl, F. "Adjustment of Displaced Persons". *Jewish Social Service Quarterly*, 1948 25, 254.

ISOLATION

We now come to a form of deprivation that is essentially psychological, that is to say the effect on the individual of separation from parents or loved ones, either through illness or through death.

The Effect of Maternal Deprivation. The effect of maternal deprivation has been a subject which has been persistently studied over a number of years. One of the first investigations was made by Goldfarb[44] who studied two main groups of children: children who had passed some part of their lives in an institution and then passed on to foster homes, and children who had lived part of their lives in their own homes before being sent to a foster home. His general conclusion was to the effect that infants who were brought up in institutions have an isolation type of experience, which had as its result an isolation type of personality. This was characterised by unsocial behaviour, aggression, insecurity and a lack of patterns for giving and receiving affection. Institution children as a group show aggressive, restless and uncontrolled behaviour, together with a retardation of language development. An important finding was that when institutionalised children were later transferred to home life, they were not able to take full advantage of this, if they were over the age of three when it occurred. Another study by the same writer made the discovery that institutionalised children have a lack of abstract thinking, because in the very early years they have not had the chance of learning with a mother figure with whom the child could identify. Goldfarb's and others' studies indicate quite clearly that the lack of a mother in the early years of life has a traumatic effect on the intellectual and personality facets of the child which have a lasting quality. How lasting this can be is indicated by the researches of Bowlby, the most prominent name in this field. In his work on stealing[45] he investigated the fact which careful enquiries had already shown, that there was a high proportion of juvenile thieves who had never lived securely in one home all their lives but had in fact spent long periods away from their home. He took as his

[44] Goldfarb, W. "Infant Rearing and Problem behavior". *Amer. J. Orthopsych.* 1943, *13*, 249. "The Effects of early institutional care on adolescent personality". *J. Exper. Educ.* 1943, *12*, 106.
[45] Bowlby, J. *Forty-four Juvenile Thieves.* 1946 Ballière.

sample forty-four consecutive cases seen at the London Child Guidance Clinic between 1936 and 1939, in whom stealing was a definite symptom. He submitted these young thieves into character types, following a psychiatric examination; the majority of the children falling into what he called the affectionless character. These were children characterised by lack of normal affection, shame or sense of responsibility. He contrasted the delinquent group with a control group of forty-four children attending the clinic but who did not steal, and who fell within the same range of age and intelligence. Results concerning causative factors at play were grouped into possible genetic factors, early home environment and contemporary environment. Of these the second factor, broken homes and separation of the child from the mother showed the biggest contrast. About forty per cent of the delinquent group had suffered an early and prolonged separation from the mother, whilst only five per cent of the control group had similarly suffered. Of the affectionless characters, eighty-five per cent had had an early separation, as compared with seventeen per cent of the other thieves in the remaining character categories. He noted further that the affectionless character was dominated by fantasies which were perpetuated by prolonged separation.

In his report to the World Health Organisation Bowlby[46] summarised the research into the effects of deprivation of this nature. He states that there is plenty of evidence to indicate that it can have harmful effects on children's development during the period of separation itself, during the period immediately after a restoration to maternal care, and permanently. As to the time in which deprivation is especially harmful there is some conflict of views. However Bowlby concludes that "For the present . . . it may be recorded that deprivation occurring in the second half of the first year of life is agreed by all students of the subject to be of great significance and that many believe this to be true also of deprivation occurring in the first half, especially from three to six months. The balance of opinion, indeed, is that considerable damage to mental health can be done by deprivation in these months, a view which is unquestionably supported by the direct observations . . . of the immediately adverse effects of deprivation on babies of this age."

[46] Bowlby, J. *Maternal Care and Mental Health*. World Health Organisation 1951 Monograph Series No. 2.

Motivation

Social Work and Separation from the Mother. Such is the general
background of the importance of early separation from the mother.
From the point of view of social workers Cram[47] has indicated
four aspects of separation which they should study, apart from
the question of hospital visiting. The four aspects she mentions
are the question at what age a baby should be adopted, the problems around the necessity of keeping a child in constant touch
with its mother if there has to be a temporary separation, the
difficult question as to whether it is worse for children to be
physically neglected or removed from a neglectful mother, and
the general problem as to what can be done to prevent the misery
of children where separation is inevitable but not complete. It
remains to be emphasised that this is a field of study to which the
student of social work should not only pay especial attention, not
only attempt to make systematic observation if there is sufficient
opportunity, but also to try and formulate fruitful hypotheses
which can be tested out by those most qualified to do so.

Enough has been said to show that the emotional attitude of the
mother and the lack of one altogether have serious consequences
on the child. It is therefore a difficult question when one is faced
with the choice of foster homes. We have already noticed some of
the motivational features of foster parents. Now we have to face
the worker's particular task of judging the influence on the child of
the foster mother and related conditions. As Deming[48] says this is
a most difficult problem and impossible to solve with any degree
of accuracy. "At best she sees the home and members of the
family two or three times before placement is made. Even if she
is extremely acute in her judgement she may have missed some
factor which turns up only after the child, with his difficulties, is
put in place as the other side of the equation." The subject of
foster placement has been brought in at this point as pointing to
the possibility of either avoiding or compensating for, maternal
deprivation. One evil, however, should not be avoided at the
expense of another evil, that is of a hasty or incorrect foster
placement. The effects of privation may well be preferable to the
choice of ill-fitted parents. Also there is the open problem of how

[47] Cram, O. W. "The separation of young children from their mothers". *Social
Work* 1949, *6*, 319.
[48] Deming, J. "Foster home and Group Placement". *Amer. J. Orthopsychiatry.*
1940, *10*, 586.

much damage may be done by the experiment of fostering following institutional life.

Conclusion. The conclusions reached by the investigators of the effect of maternal deprivation should be tempered with one or two modifications. Not every child who has been separated from or lost its mother in early life becomes delinquent or shows some other undesirable characteristic. Conversely not every delinquent has lost his mother. Researches into this question may suffer from the drawback of the samples being highly selective. Nevertheless it is a factor of the highest importance and further work on the subject may clarify the position.[49]

[49] Other writings should be consulted for an evaluation of the maternal deprivation hypothesis. Thus Lewis, H. *Deprived Children*, O.U.P. 1954, while not wholly disagreeing with the main hypothesis does emphasise factors other than maternal separation which influence mental ill-health. The "affectionless" character was found, in this sample, to have no particular relationship to being separated from his or her mother. A more direct negation that Bowlby's thesis has been established is to be found in a full summary of the available evidence made by O'Connor, N. "The evidence for the permanently disturbing effects of mother child separation." *Acta Psychologica* 1956, *12*, 174.

III

LEARNING

THIS subject, inasmuch as it is contained in the term learning theory, has become the central topic of the leading psychologists in the last generation or so. Beginning with an interest in animal psychology it has irradiated to become a means of constructing systems that are, in their way, as methodologically satisfactory as anything in the natural sciences. Logical constructs are built up and able to be put to the experimental test. The intention behind this line of psychological enquiry is to create a science of behaviour which is strictly experimental, and which will contain theories that can hold or fall with putting them to the test. One of the more convenient ways of doing this is to employ animals under laboratory conditions, as the fundamental processes of learning and behaviour are more easily seen in organisms that are lower down the evolutionary scale than man, and which are more amenable to experimental intereference. This does not necessarily mean that we can predict straightaway the behaviour of a man from the behaviour of a rat; rather it means that those mechanisms which are in man, complicated by the higher intellectual processes, are seen more clearly in the behaviour of the animal. Therefore a close and detailed investigation of the laws operating behind the animal's behaviour should help us to understand the basic human principles of behaviour.

It would be outside the scope of this volume to indicate in any detail the theories and controversies that have arisen in this area of psychology; the intention is only to introduce basic concepts and definitions, to delineate the main types of learning and to touch on a few eminent theories.

DEFINITION

Learning should be distinguished from maturation. There are

certain activities which are inherited by the organisation and development of the body. Not only is the internal regulation of the body not learned but activities such as reaching, sitting up, standing and walking are primarily dependent on the growth patterns of the organism. When these patterns have reached a certain stage, then the activity which belongs to them is manifested. And although they may be delayed or promoted by external methods, they are not dependent upon them. So that there is a range of modifications which cannot be said to be learned but is the result of maturation. So the term "learning" is reserved for that class of activity through which the individual modifies his behaviour, and which cannot be attributed to processes identifiable to the growth of the body. As a matter of fact it is not so simple a matter to give a clear-cut definition as there is often a mixture of maturation and learning proper. Nevertheless, the definition given by Hilgard[1] indicates the differentiation: "Learning is the process by which an activity originates or is changed through training procedures (whether in the laboratory or in the natural environment) as distinguished from changes by factors not attributable to training." In this category, then, is included a host of activities such as swimming, dancing, driving a car, reading and writing, as well as the more complex process of learning to adapt to society.

TYPES

There is some speculation and controversy as to whether there is fundamentally only one type of learning, or two types, or several. We shall not concern outselves at this level, but merely outline some of the types of learning that are known.

Conditioning. The conditioned response is no doubt the most simple of learned activities. It results from a persistence of associations between one activity and another. For example, I take a medicine that is abhorrent to me, and I express distaste. Now if I see the medicine bottle often enough when I taste the liquid in it, then after a number of such "pairings", the mere sight of the bottle is sufficient to create an expression of distaste. Bernard Shaw[2] tells of an example of a conditioned reflex when visiting

[1] Hilgard, E. R. *Theories of Learning.* Appleton-Century-Crofts 1948.
[2] Shaw, G. B. *Everybody's Political What's What?* Constable 1944.

a naval exhibition at Chelsea. "In the passage between the P. and O. cabins I suddenly felt seasick, and had to beat a hasty retreat into the gardens. This was a perfect example of a conditioned reflex. I had often been made seasick by the rolling and pitching of a ship. The rolling and pitching had been accompanied by the sight of the passengers' quarters and the smell of paint and oakum. The connection between them had been so firmly established in me that even when I stood on the firm earth these sights and smells made me squeamish."

Although everyday life presents numerous examples of conditioned responses, the concept was only firmly established at the beginning of the century by Pavlov.[3] Experimenting with dogs, Pavlov found that if there was a stimulus frequently associated with the presentation of food, the display of the stimulus alone would have the same effect on the animal as the food. Food in the mouth elicits salivation, secretion of the salivary gland. When a bell (if it is an auditory stimulus) is paired with the food, then after a while the sounding of the bell alone will cause salivation. In other words the nervous system of the animal has become accustomed to connect the sound of a bell with the sight and taste of food. When the bell is sounded alone (without the food) the organism responds in a manner appropriate to the advent of food. In the technical language that Pavlov employed, the taste of food in the mouth was the unconditioned stimulus and the response that it elicited (salivation) was the unconditioned response. The hitherto neutral stimulus (the bell) was labelled the conditioned stimulus and the almost similar response of salivation and expectant attitude of the animal was called the conditioned response. The words "almost similar" are used because the animal does not go through the mime of eating when there is no food. There are some addenda to this simple situation of conditioning that are important to note. The first is that there can be a generalisation of stimuli that are conditioned. One of the earliest behaviourists conditioned fear in a child by presenting a white rat and a loud noise. Very soon the mere sight of the white rat alone caused fear. Now it was found that not only the white rat did this but also a white rabbit and a white dog. There was a generalisation from the original stimulus of the rat. Alternatively it is possible to train an animal to be conditioned to certain

[3] Pavlov, I. P. *Conditioned Reflexes.* O.U.P. 1927.

stimuli and not to others. For example it might be possible to set up conditioning by presenting a hundred watt bulb with the food, and not present food with a fifty watt bulb. Salivation will then be effected with the brighter light and not with the dimmer one. This is known as differentiation of stimuli. This brings us to the point that the neutral stimulus must be "reinforced". For Pavlov found that when the conditioned stimulus was presented alone there was a gradual fading of the conditioned response. Again in technical terms the response is said to be "extinguished". In the classical laboratory situation experimental extinction is effected by presenting the bell alone for a number of times without any food.

"Social" Conditioning. Such is the laboratory picture of conditioning. In everyday life there are not only examples of the order of associating taste with the sight of a bottle, there are also more important instances where social values and attitudes are likewise conditioned. It is interesting to speculate how far conditioning is possible through the media of films, newspapers and radio. Huxley's *Brave New World* and Orwell's *Nineteen Eighty-Four* give fictitious examples of what it would be like if our social valuations were rigidly conditioned by an omnipotent State system. Yet even in our own society it is questionable how far racial prejudice is a matter of conditioning. The sight of a black skin (say) paired with a frequent disapproving gesture and spoken comment by parents may create an attitude towards negroes which may be continually "reinforced" by the whole social mileau of the child throughout the impressionable years. And this is an attitude which becomes so encrusted in the personality of the individual that no simple method of extinction by verbal means is possible to shift.

Trial and Error. The origin of this type of learning lay in the early experiments of Thorndike[4] with cats in puzzle-boxes. He placed the cat in a cage with a latch which could be simply operated by the animal, and placed some food outside the cage. The problem for the cat was merely to open the cage and thus get at the food. Thorndike showed, by means of this simple situation, that the animal hit upon the correct method of release by a process of

[4] Thorndike, E. L. *Animal Intelligence* 1911.

trial and error. Thus at the first instance the cat released the catch accidentally, possibly by rubbing against it. At the second test it takes less time to do this until finally there comes the trial when it goes straight to the latch and lets itself out. As Thorndike pointed out this type of behaviour is characterised by selection and connection. The animal puts together in a sequence a number of appropriate acts and selects the ones that fit the problem. Only this is a gradual process and there is no sudden solution. As a matter of fact later experiments have questioned the assumption that Thorndike's cats were behaving as randomly as was thought, yet again everyday experience seems to suggest, on the surface at any rate, that quite a large amount of our own experience is built up in this fashion. However one of the more important pronouncements of this school of learning was the formulation of the law of effect. This principle said that those responses of the animal that were followed by satisfaction tended to become more strengthened, those responses that were followed by dissatisfaction tended to become weakened. Attention to the consequences of learning thus placed motivation very much into the picture, and it is important enough to warrant a later sub-section to the subject.

"Insight". Quite a different type of learning was demonstrated by Köhler, in his work with the higher primates.[5] A typical experiment was to place a chimpanzee in a cage with two sticks which could be joined together. A banana was put outside the cage, out of range of one stick but capable of being drawn in with combination of the two sticks. Close observation of the behaviour of the chimpanzee with the two sticks made it appear that the animal suddenly grasped the solution of the problem. There appeared to be no trial and error conduct; the animal behaved in what we would call an intelligent manner, in a way that was insightful. Further variants of the initial experiment were performed by creating obstacles to the procurement of the fruit, or dangling the banana on the top of the cage so that the chimpanzee had to put two or more boxes on top of one another in order to reach it. Solution of all these problems showed that insight was the predominating mechanism. The animal seemed to grasp the idea of the problem. In everyday life a mundane example of

[5] Köhler, W. *The Mentality of Apes.* London 1925.

insight is suddenly seeing the solution of a crossword clue. Creative work no doubt works on a very similar principle. Perhaps it is mathematicians who shows this type of learning most clearly. Scientists such as Poincare, Gauss and Einstein[6] have all written about the sudden solution of a problem about which they had been concerned, and which suddenly came "out of the blue" to them. Described in this way, of course, insight is analogous to intuition and is a far cry from experiments with animals. Only the latter type of example is peculiarly human and should not be neglected in considering insightful behaviour.

LEARNING AND MOTIVATION

We have already remarked that in conditioning, the hitherto neutral stimulus must be "reinforced" by food, in order that the sequence be maintained. In other words the food acted as a reward. Now there is some disagreement in learning theory as to whether reinforcement is a logical necessity for learning to take place, but whatever the outcome may be of this controversy, there is little doubt that the relationship between learning and motivation is of importance. This can be seen in a celebrated experiment by Abel,[7] who asked a group of sixty boys to solve a finger maze. Evenly matched for age and intelligence, he split the children up into three groups, the first of which he gave no reward at all for having solved the maze, the second being given a penny (material reward) and the third receiving social recognition—a verbal reward of "Good" or "Very good". The no-reward group not only learned the task more slowly than the others but also made the largest amount of errors. The verbal reward group made less errors and learned faster than the no-reward group, yet slower than the material reward boys, who also made the least mistakes.

Reinforcement, of course, depends upon motivation in the first place. If an animal is not hungry the acquirement of food is no reward at all. If there is motivation, however, the factor of reinforcement acts as a selective agent in the learning task. Those activities that are rewarded will be learned, those that are not rewarded tend not to be learned so well. It might be mentioned

[6] See Beveridge, W. I. B. *The Art of Scientific Investigation.* Heinemann 1951.
[7] Abel, L. B. "The effects of shift in motivation upon the learning of a sensori-motor task". *Arch. Psychol.* 1936, 205. A "finger-maze" is performed blindfolded.

in passing that the role of punishment, so far as can be seen from the experimental literature, does not act in the negative direction with as much force as reward does in the positive. That is to say, learned acts are not eliminated effectively by the application of punishment. It may suppress a response but not necessarily weaken the bonds of a learned act.[8]

Turning from the laboratory conditions of learning theory to conditions of everyday life, it is worth while pointing out that the notion of what constitutes a reward can be very different for people. Some "bad habits" and "ways of life" are adopted because they are found rewarding. Teddy-boys stand on street-corners because they find it rewarding, and any middle-class club-leader who thinks his club would be "just the thing" for them forgets that what *he* finds rewarding is not regarded as such at all by the teddy-boy. What is necessary to find out in such cases is exactly what is the motivating influence at work that is rewarded in this fashion.

HABITS

It is a common adage that we are all creatures of habit. By this is meant that we acquire patterns of behaviour which have been learned in relation to some situation, and which are thereafter performed repetitively. For example, we learn to use the typewriter in a certain way, depending very largely on the combination of numerous finger movements. In the beginning, as with all skills, there is difficulty in applying the fingers to the appropriate keys. After a while there is no more need for a conscious effort; the fingers appear to find their own way to the keys, and in fact, as in the case of a housewife knitting to "music while you work", it is quite possible to perform a skill adequately while paying attention to something else entirely. The word "habit" with its adjective "habitual" is given to this phenomenon. This does not explain it, it only gives a label to it. To say that some sequence is habitual is only to say that it has become repetitive and relatively autonomous. It does not tell us why this is so.

---

[8] For the role of punishment in learning see Bugelski, B. R. *The Psychology of Learning*. Methuen 1956 Chapter 10. For a detailed summary of the controversies in learning theory see Spence, K. W. "Theoretical Interpretations of Learning". in S. S. Stevens: *Handbook of Experimental Psychology*. Wiley 1951.

Explanation would consist of the analysis of a habit, the mechanism of it, possibly depending on an extension of the conditioned reflex concept,[9] although it is considered by many that the conditioned response is not adequate to fulfil the mechanism of habit.

Habit and Motivation. In his *Talks to Teachers on Psychology*,[10] William James in a characteristic phrase spoke of mankind being a "bundle of habits" and declared that "ninety-nine hundredths or, possibly, nine hundred and ninety-nine thousandths of our activity is purely automatic and habitual, from our rising in the morning to our lying down each night." And although the rather rigid conception of a habit, noted by James, as being the end result of a series of muscular contractions has been disfavoured to the notion of habit being infinitely more plastic, there is still much in James's argument that a very great deal of our actions are habitual. The idea, however, of habit being merely a matter of use or disuse, in the same sort of way that the grooves in a gramophone record are rendered deeper with the continued playing of it, has been considered by many learning theorists as faulty, without considering the facts of motivation and reward. In fact it is able to be demonstrated experimentally that the remark made by one of the gentlemen of Verona (Valentine) that "use doth breed a habit in a man!" is downright wrong. Though as a matter of fact the ensuing lines

' This shadowy desert, unfrequented woods,
I better brook than flourishing peopled towns ',

show that reinforcement for Valentine consisted of being alone in the forest away from the hurly burly of urban life. It was not the fact that he had done this in the past that made it a habit for this Shakespearean character, but the fact that his temperament preferred it.

In short, although repetition or usage enters into the formation of a habit, it has been argued that it is not dependent upon these alone, but upon the needs of an organism and upon the satisfaction of these needs.

[9] See Humphrey, G. "Is the conditioned reflex the unit of habit?" *J. Abn. and Soc. Psychol.* 1925, *20*, 10.
[10] James, W. *Talks to Teachers on Psychology.* Longmans 1900.

FORMATION

We have already seen that there is some controversy as to whether the conditioned reflex is the unit of habit or not. The range of habits is too complex to be built up from a series of conditioned responses. It is possible, however, to outline the stages in the establishment of a habit. Koerth[11] distinguishes three steps: that of having a clear image or idea of the movement or act to be attained, that of an analysis of the various activities involved, and thirdly that of the repetition of the series of acts. As Koerth points out there are many habits formed without a clear idea of the end to be reached, but the habit is better inculcated by so having it. Analysis means essentially a process of selection, leaving out those acts which are unnecessary for or uneconomical to the sequence, and reinforcing those which are directly appropriate. Repetition is a practice which continually strengthens the habit, although we tend to think of it more in connection with physiological or motor habits rather than those of an emotional nature.

Principles from Learning Theory. There are two principles which have originated in the learning theory of Clerk Hull[12] and which have been tested in the laboratory with the maze habits of rats, that may be generalised to human situations. The first is the hypothesis of the goal gradient. By this was meant that there was a certain underlying connection between a learner and the goal he was approaching. This connection was in the form of a gradient such that the nearer the learner approached the goal the stronger would be the power evoked by it. Putting this into the practical situations of the experiments performed by this school, it meant that, on this hypothesis, the rat would be expected to run faster as the goal was being approached than at the beginning of the maze; responses which were near the goal would be conditioned more strongly than those far removed from it; and blind alleys in the maze would be eliminated by the animal far more quickly at the end of the maze than those at the beginning. It is as though the animal puts on a spurt, both physically and intellectually, when the end is perceived. Let us take an everyday habit which might

[11] Koerth, W. "Control Through Habits", Chapter IV of Starch D. and others *Controlling Human Behavior.* MacMillan 1938.

[12] The original formulations are in Hull, C. L. "The Goal Gradient hypothesis and maze learning". *Psychol. Review* 1932, *39*, 25 and "The concept of the habit-family hierarchy and maze learning". *Psychol. Review* 1934, *41*, 33 & 134.

bring out this idea. Suppose that a person is in the habit of going to a certain restaurant every day at eleven to take a coffee. When he sets out he may make a number of unnecessary circumnavigations; as he approaches the restaurant he proceeds more directly and goes straight to the shop. Once in the restaurant his actions become more conditioned by the surroundings. The ways of ordering a coffee are limited and his actions are more directly appropriate to the drinking of this beverage. To be sure it is by no means a simple matter to transfer the experiments with rats over to the situations of people in everyday life. As has been noticed previously, the complexities of human actions mask the mechanisms of learning which are more easily observable with organisms of a simpler nature. Neverthless concepts such as the ones we are discussing can be referred to our own behaviour as long as the complexity is held in mind.

The second principle which Hull enunciates is what he termed the habit family hierarchy. There are always a number of alternative routes between a starting point and the goal. These alternatives are integrated into a family, that is to say they are all mutually related by virtue of their origin and by their end, the starting-point and the goal. But it is a family in which there is order. For it is clear, taking the idea of reinforcement into account, that some alternatives are more strongly conditioned to the goal than to others. To take our example of the coffee again; to choose a table at which a waiter was serving would be more strongly linked with the ultimate goal—the drinking of the coffee—than choosing a table at which no service was given. In short there will be preferred routes and preferred means, the preference depending upon the appropriateness of attaining the goal. Routes and means which are less favoured would only be chosen when the preferred ones are blocked. The next appropriate ones would then be selected. If there was no service at our restaurant then the preferred table would be the one nearest the exit of the self-service counter, and so forth.

These principles of Hull seem far removed from the way in which we usually think about our habits, and it may be inadvisable to take them out of their system context. We only do this in order to attempt to provide a customary application of a prominent branch of theoretical psychology, and to stress that, complex though they may be, human actions may have underlying principles of explanation no less than for the rat. The question as to whether *these* are the appropriate explanations is another matter. They are given as one example of the laws underlying learning, which together make up habit systems.

SOCIAL FUNCTION

A great deal of what are termed social habits is considered in contemporary psychology under the heading of "Attitudes", a subject which will be discussed seaparately in the following Section. Over one generation ago John Dewey[13] thought of habit as an all-important factor in the study of social psychology. "In addition to the general psychology of habit . . . we need to find out just how different customs shape the desires, beliefs, purposes of those who are affected by them. The problem of social psychology is not how either individual or collective mind forms social groups and customs, but how different customs, established interacting arrangements, form and nurture different minds." And later, ". . . the forming of habits becomes a guarantee for the maintenance of hedges of custom." As Allport remarks,[14] Dewey attempted to give far too much latitude to the term, and his concept of it was consequently vague. But Dewey's contribution was noteworthy in emphasising the elaborate system of habits prevalent in a society which have social relevance. The insistence on social habits is very largely an outcome of the controversy between the ideas of the relative importance of heredity and environment (see the Section in the Chapter on Personality). The argument has been between patterns of instinct and learned sets of behaviour. Habit has thus become to be regarded as the antithesis of the instinct doctrine.

The social function of habits may be thought of as twofold. There is the economy of learning, and repetitively reinforcing, a set of beliefs or customs which are economical and of utility value. If we can regard as a social habit the regulation of always stopping at the red colour of traffic lights, then it is clear that this is a convention which saves much time and energy for all concerned, and is useful in saving deaths. Teaching the individual at an early age to regard with respect the red lights is a social device that

[13] Dewey, J. *Human Nature and Conduct.* Holt 1922.
[14] Allport, G. W. "The Historical background of modern social Psychology". In Lindzey, G. *Handbook of Social Psychology.* Vol. I. Addison-Wesley Publishing Co. 1954.

has some value. The other social function consists in the trans-mission of cultural traits, from one generation to another, which uphold the tradition of that culture. For example, in our own society it has become habitual for the husband to go out to work while the wife looks after the children and home. This is a custom which the child comes to apprehend in its formative years and regard as habitual. But there are certain cultures where the opposite takes place, and in fact even in our own society (and certainly in contemporary American life), this particular habit is breaking down. The social habit is changing. Change though it may, the point is that many customs, such as this one, tend to be regarded as a feature of society, and are strengthened by a con-tinuity of attitude. Thus this second function of habits is a bolstering of conventions. When the habits break down, then there is to be expected a modification of the convention.

HABIT AND PERSONALITY

There is a well-known story about Kant to the effect that his neighbours would set their clocks by his daily afternoon walk, and whatever this anecdote enlightens us about the speculations of the German philosopher, it implies still more that it was a part of Kant's personality to be so methodical. Methodicality and the individual Immanuel Kant went hand in hand. It was a permanent trait in this philosopher. Such examples could be multiplied, both for famous people and for one's own acquaintances. In fact there are many persons in whom a habitual trait is so dominant that they are remembered for that alone. Uriah Heep is remembered for his mock humility, while to judge from contemporary interest, Davy Crockett would seem to be best remembered for his head-wear. The latter may be a trivial and flippant example; it serves to remind us however that habitual mannerisms, gestures, ways of dress, postures, turns of speech and mental outlook, together make up a picture of a personality which is readily identifiable. In fact we are wont to say when a friend departs from his custom-ary manner that "so-and-so was not himself today". Moreover it is a reflection of the interaction between personality and social environment that such a habitual feature as a gesture can be modified under a fresh impact of a new society.[15]

[15] See Efron, D. and Foley, J. P. Jnr. "Gestural behavior and Social Setting". In Newcomb, T. M. and Hartley, E. L. *Readings in Social Psychology*. Holt 1947.

Habit, then, must be considered as a component of personality. The extreme form of this viewpoint has come to regard personality as habit adjustment. Guthrie, who has emphasised the importance of association in learning, maintains this outlook as follows:[16] "Mental life consists in adjusting to recurring change by changes in the behavior of the organism itself. And since by personality we mean the stable behavior of the organism, this consists largely of adjustive changes and *can be well described in terms of the world that is adjusted to.*" Guthrie continues to state that if we know what sort of world the individual inhabits, we can tell in advance many of the traits he will develop without examining him. Not all of the theorists of personality formation would go the whole way with Guthrie on this, nor would it be maintained generally that personality is synonymous with habit adjustment. The thesis, though, does help to bring out a point which is often forgotten, namely that what the layman regards as a recognisable trait of personality is in fact a well-established system of habits.

As against this notion we have the viewpoint expressed by Allport in his treatment of the theory of identical elements.[17] He takes the example of courtesy: under the identical element theory, courtesy is regarded as a repetition of a series of habits (taking off a cap to a woman for example) stimulated by a situation which had been previously associated with it. Allport, however, then treats courtesy as a trait of a higher order than a specific habit, or a bundle of them. Specific habits are generalised with development and replaced in time by traits. Habits, so to speak, would be at the command of the trait, which is regarded by the individual as an ideal of conduct. Allport continues with his example of courtesy to say that if a youth was transported to China, most of his habits associated with courtesy would require readjustment. This would be effected and yet still consistent with his ideal. Thus, on this showing habit is recognised as being a component of personality, but is denied the status of a "nothing-but" outlook. It is relegated to a lower position in a hierarchy in which traits and types would be higher.

This viewpoint fits in better with the current conception of a habit that is plastic and variant. This does not mean that some

---

[16] Guthrie, E. R. "Personality in terms of Associative Learning". In J. M. Hunt: *Personality and the Behaviour Disorders*. Ronald 1944. Vol. I.

[17] Allport, G. W. *Personality*. Constable 1937.

habits may not become separated from the total mass of personality and behave autonomously. It means that it is not sufficient to regard the complex structure of personality in this way, although it is valuable to take habit into account as a part.

ATTITUDES

As was explained in the previous section, the study and concept of attitudes has superseded that which used to be discussed under the heading of social habits. In ordinary language one tends to speak of attitude in one of two ways. We use the term in the sense of a posture or pose—"he struck an attitude of defiance". Or we use the word in a way which suggests that there is something underlying a person's visible actions, which influences them. The King in *Through the Looking-Glass* uses the term in the first way, when in response to Alice's observation that the messenger exhibited curious behaviour (he was skipping up and down and wriggling like an eel) answers: "Not at all. He's an Anglo-Saxon Messenger—and those are Anglo-Saxon attitudes". When we talk about "dumb insolence", that is to say when a person *seems* to be rude without actually expressing it in speech (an offence in the Navy), we are using the term in the second way. In the history of psychology, these two ways have been used by writers in much the same fashion, namely motor and mental attitudes. What is implied is that there is a pre-disposing outlook, a tendency to do this or that (or not do this or that), a tendency which is not manifest itself but which induces this or that behaviour to be shown. The phrase "state of readiness" is often used to define an attitude, indicating that the organism is in a state which can respond to certain situations and will if they arise.[18]

Types of Attitudes. Everybody has various attitudes about their beliefs, about their actions, about other people's beliefs and actions, and about abstract questions in addition. Thus we come to talk about political, racial and religious attitudes, meaning

---

[18] The term attitude has tended also to replace that of *sentiment* which was associated with earlier psychologists such as Shand and McDougall. Albeit there are some differences between the two terms, although exact clarification is lacking. Broadly speaking a sentiment is an emotional disposition, centred around a concrete object and generally considered to be more lasting and more organised than an attitude. Patriotism can be considered as an example.

that not only do we have ideas and beliefs about these matters, but meaning that our particular conduct in questions of importance regarding them are swayed by the attitude we hold about them. A person who believes in *Apartheid* is likely to take a characteristic point of view to all matters involving colour and the rights of black folk, and would be expected to show actions which would be consistent with this belief. The importance of studies on attitude, whether they are conscious or unconscious, cannot be exaggerated. A man's beliefs and actions are not completely piecemeal; they are given some measure of continuity by the social attitudes which he takes, or which are enforced upon him by the social climate in which he lives. The social psychologist or social scientist when he moves in realms affected by the psychology of the people involved, has to reckon in a very practical way with individual and group attitudinal traits. The social worker, when he or she deals with a client has to confront not only the views and problems which are demonstrated; he or she also has to calculate with the *undisclosed* opinions which are the individual items of a generalised outlook. A knowledge of the attitude which a person has on any particular subject, or indeed to life in general, helps us to assess his particular remarks and actions in the light of it.

DEVELOPMENT

The child acquires a number of appropriate social skills and habits from its own family, relationships with other children, from school and other sources. We must now dwell on the development of those constellations of social habits that we call attitudes, and enquire how it is that a child comes to hold this or that attitude.

The answer is not so simple and explanatory as may at first appear. There has been no *exact* study of the way in which infants and children do in fact acquire attitudes. What is clear is the general outline. Thus, as Newcomb[19] points out, in the early stages of attitudinal development there is no sharp differentiation between individual attitudes. ". . . one favorable attitude is very much like another, and all unfavorable attitudes are much alike." Newcomb considers attitudes to be developed from a generalising of drives which are learned by experience. A child acquires a

[19] Newcomb, T. M. *Social Psychology.* Tavistock 1950.

preferred taste for sweets: he learns by experience that sweets are attained through a devious route of mother, money and sweet-shop. In this manner, what commenced as an agreeable taste is generalised into an attitude favourable to the various means of appeasing that taste. The word "sweet-shop" evokes a similar reaction. In this way there is built up an edifice of a characteristic type. Later stages make the whole system considerably more complex, and there are created integrations and hierarchies of attitudes. That is to say certain attitudes become joined with others, and they are connected into one integrated piece. Some attitudes are quite evidently stronger than others. One single attitude may become a leit-motif throughout a person's entire life, colouring all his actions.

Formation of Social Attitudes. The formation of attitudes is the result of an amalgamation of personal temperament and social influences, and although each person has a different and possibly unique organisation of them, it becomes apparent that there are representative types of attitudes that can be attached either to temperament, on the one hand, or to social issues on the other. Authorities like Sherif[20] have emphasised the social issues, although he recognises that not all an individual's attitudes are social. His standpoint is revealed when he states that "attitudes are formed in relation to situations, persons or groups with which the individual comes into contact in the course of his development. Once formed, they demand that the individual react in a *characteristic* way to these or related situations, persons, or groups." It is of course obvious that the very term "attitude" precludes it arising in a vacuum. There has to be an attitude toward somebody or something. From the developmental aspect, interest is orientated towards the people and situations which help to form the attitude. As might be expected, to be in a position to study this observationally is no easy matter. However Horowitz and Horowitz[21] managed to observe the development of social attitudes in children in process. The particular attitudes studied were those relating towards sex, age, and race, particularly the attitude towards Negroes. (The children studied belonged to a

[20] Sherif, M. *An Outline of Social Psychology*. Harper 1948.
[21] Horowitz, E. L. and R. E. "Development of social attitudes in children". *Sociometry* 1938, *1*, 301.

small rural community in the American South). The authors make it clear that the attitude towards negroes appears to have its origin with the parents of the child. We shall see later that there is evidence that there is not always a correlation between parents and children in this respect, but this does not affect the present issue of the origin of an attitude. In the author's own words: "the children develop their attitudes, at first quite well aware of their sources, but toward adolescence tending to lose conscious recollection of these origins, devise rationalisation of various sorts to support them, and maintain them little changed." It is commented, however, that there is some evidence to the suggestion that qualitative changes do occur in the course of development. These are related to the development of the personality organisation and structure. This brings us back to a former point, namely that attitudes as such are a mixture of the influences coming from temperament and the influences which a person meets as these develop. The various combinations of these two influences are of course immense, and it is only when we can generalise in a large embrace of attitudes, as when we talk of a "conservative" attitude can we hope to sort them out in origin.

METHODS

It becomes necessary at this point to dwell a moment on the subject of attitude research, on the means whereby psychologists ascertain the vouchsafed attitudes of men, women and children. It is unnecessary to go very fully into this, particularly as there exists convenient summaries on the subject.[22]

Scales. We recall that attitudes are inferred from a person's behaviour; in technical language they are "hypothetical variables". That is to say, for explanatory purposes a factor which is not directly observable has to be supposed in order to account for the visible happenings. Now attitudes are measured by a scaling procedure on the basis of either questionnaires or interviews. The scale is such that it measures the order of preference or non-preference, favourableness or unfavourableness, to the attitude being measured. We are all familiar with physical scales, such as the ruler, vernier and thermometer. They differ in their construction and range of measurability, but they all have in common an order

[22] See for example, Sprott, W. J. H. *Social Psychology*. Methuen 1952 Ch. VII.

of numerical positions. In psychological scales there is the same principle, except that individuals are assigned to particular positions along the scale. Also psychological scales are generally interested in the *relative* degree of an attitude. In other words that which can be measured in respect, say, to the attitude towards Jews is only that Mr. X dislikes Jews *more* than Mr. Y and *less* than Mr. Z. There is nothing in the nature of a "boiling point" or a "freezing point" (except in a metaphorical sense) in attitudes to which we might have any absolute values. As in physical science there are different sorts of scales, constructed differently. There is for example the social-distance scale, as originated by Bogardus.[23] Essentially this is a device to measure the social acceptability of a nationality group. The scale is constructed from a number of items in a questionnaire. The person who fills out the questionnaire is required to answer questions which aim at the extent to which he will accept or not accept nationality groups other than his own. For example there is an order of acceptability ranging from a willingness to accept the different nationality group (English, French, Chinese, Negro, Russian, Turks etc.) as a member of one's own family through marriage, through such classification as willingness to accept "to my club as personal chums" and "to employment in my occupation", to the degree, lowest in the series, of complete non-acceptability, "would exclude from my country". There are seven such classifications on the scale, and all that the subject is required to do is to indicate which of the seven points he would choose in relation to the nationality group. The results thus give a relative picture of nationality preferences. On such a scale one can say that an Englishman who answers the questions may place high in the series Americans, Frenchmen and Swedes, but put low in the series Greeks and Russians. This only tells us that the first three nationalities are preferred more than the last three. It cannot tell to what extent more, because there is no qualification on such a scale that the intervals between the points are equal. To remedy such an obvious limitation Thurstone[24] constructed an attitude scale by the method of equal-appearing intervals. In this method the difficulty of judging the distance between points is surmounted

[23] Bogardus, E. S. "A Social Distance Scale". *Sociology and Social Research.* 1933, 17, 265.

[24] Thurstone, L. and Chave, E. J. *The Measurement of Attitudes.* Univ. Chicago Press 1929.

by having a large number of judges, working independently of one another, sort hundreds of statements related to the attitude in question into a number of piles, ranging from most favourable to the next favourable to the one after next favourable and so on down to the least favourable. The value on the scale to which a particular statement is given depends on the middlemost value to which the whole group of judges has given it. All this is done in the stage of construction before the questions are given to the subject, and of course the latter does not know the actual scale values of the items he is answering. All that he has to do is to tick off a statement with which he agrees. If there is a statement to the effect that coloured people are lazy and should only be given menial jobs in the community, and he agrees with this, all that he has to do on the form is to tick it.

A limitation of the above two scales is that they represent an "all or none" attitude. Either you agree with the statement or you do not. There is no allowable *degree* of acceptability within each separate statement. Attempts to get over this difficulty are exemplified by the Likert-Type scale.[25] Here there is room for degree of approval or disapproval of a statement. The number of available degrees may vary. Some scales of this type have three, some five, others seven points. One might have on such a scale three points on a positive side such as strongly agree, moderately agree, and agree; on the negative side there are the same qualifications to the word "disagree". There would therefore be six degrees ranging from strong agreement to strong disagreement. A seventh could be inserted representing a neutral point of view, such as "undecided" or "do not know". The scale can be given numerical positions such as plus 3, plus 2 etc. through zero to minus 2 and minus 3, but it must be remembered that difficulties may arise in this. Although the difference between plus 3 and plus 2 is *arithmetically* similar to the difference between, say, zero and minus 1, there is no reason to suppose that they are *psychologically* the same. The difference between moderately approving of something and strongly approving of it cannot necessarily be equated with having an undecided attitude and expressing disagreement nor can it necessarily be equated with moderately disagreeing and strongly disagreeing. There are ways around this

[25] Likert, R. "A technique for the measurement of attitudes". *Arch. Psychol.* 1932 No. 140. See p. 152 for further remarks on rating scales.

obstacle as well as there are other methods of constructing scales, but enough has been expressed to give the general nature of the measurement of attitudes. We now turn to some of the applications.

PARENTAL ATTITUDES

The study of parental attitudes towards children, and the effects of these, has been taken up either from the angle of the result of deprivation on the children (already discussed in the previous chapter), or from the standpoint of the relationship of agreement between parents and children. Concerning the latter it has been found that there is not such a close agreement between them as might have been thought or as some early studies have borne out. Hirschberg and Gilliland,[26] for example, have qualified this assertion by discovering that parent-child correlations of attitudes differ from one kind of belief to another. They admitted that there was a relationship but that it inclined to vary according to the home situation, the subject who was tested and the actual attitude tested. Summarising this research Krech and Crutchfield[27] have said that "to say that the family is important in shaping attitudes or beliefs is not equivalent to saying that the child will take over attitudes and beliefs ready-made from the parents. The influence is possible, but whether the child will develop or not develop the same belief as his parents hold depends upon the importance and meaning of that belief for the child himself."

Reflecting on the one hand the complexity of the relationships between children and their parents, and on the other the complicated nature of attitudes, assimilating as they do the influences of many different circumstances, it is perhaps no small wonder that there is not a simple connection. It is easy to see the connection in such a broad concept as prejudice. It is not so simple to observe when it comes to attitudes of specific issues, even of prejudice toward a *particular* person. Thus a child may imbibe the general atmosphere of prejudice towards Negroes as a class and yet make an exception to those who belong to his gang.

The attitude towards authority over the child by the parents may well have a strong influence on this issue. The degree of correlation of attitudes between parents and children, in other

[26] Hirschberg, G. and Gilliland, A. R. "Parent-child relationships in attitude". *J. Abn. Soc. Psychol.* 1942, *37*, 125.

[27] Krech, D. and Crutchfield, R. S. *Theory and Problems of Social Psychology*. McGraw-Hill 1948

words, may be affected by the degree of authority with which the child is faced. It might be supposed, looking at it naively, that a rejected child will not have the same amount of agreement with its parents over some belief as a totally accepted child. Even this may not prove so simple as it might appear, as the nature of the belief itself may make a large difference, irrespective of the parental atmosphere. In the study already quoted of Hirschberg and Gilliland there was a high correlation of attitude toward the New Deal. This, as they explain, is because institutional factors affect the family as a whole, and, it might be appended, affect it irrespective of the pattern of parental authority, although this is a matter which could be settled by research. Certainly the degree of parental authority is a factor which could enter into the matter in an important way. Over and above the question of parental influence, and yet connected with it, is the matter of cultural influence. The fact that parents are involved in a network of values and customs connected with a particular culture, means that parental attitude is contingent on the cultural background.

POLITICAL AND RACIAL

One of the most paramount issues in attitude research is that of the orientation towards a definite social outlook, manifested in a political creed or nationality bias. Common observation tells us that from between the period of adolescence to the end of life, most people show some sort of behaviour which could be labelled political or racial. Again this is a subject upon which much has been written and many investigations made.[28] From a psychological point of view what is of interest is the question whether there is a connection between ideology and temperament. This question is not peculiar to psychologists of course: Sir William Gilbert may be considered to have phrased it in *Iolanthe* (often quoted in this connection) when he wrote that:

> 'I often think it's comical
> How Nature always doth contrive
> That every boy and every gal,
> That's born into the world alive,
> Is either a little Liberal,
> Or else a little Conservative.'

[28] See principally Eysenck, H. J. *The Psychology of Politics*. Routledge and Kegan Paul 1954.

Radical-Conservative Factor. What appears to have been firmly established is the existence of a political attitude known as the radical-conservative factor. This means that there are two distinct patterns, reflecting a number of diverse attitudes to personal and social affairs. Thus Eysenck has shown experimentally that opinions are not independent; they tend to collect into clusters. Opinions such as that flogging should be retained, the death penalty upheld, children should be brought up strictly, the family system should be held together, as well as a belief in private property and an adherence to orthodox religion, all go together and are viewpoints held by those people who tend to vote conservative at an election or in some way attach themselves to the Conservative creed. As against this pattern, there is the other pattern, known as the radical ideology, in which the following sets of opinions and beliefs are assembled: Anti-patriotism and anti-religious views, anti-class distinctions and in fact the very opposite of all the particular points upheld by the conservative outlook. Writing from the standpoint of psycho-analysis, Flugel[29] has designated the "right" and "left" attitudes from the aspect of identification with the parent figure, thereby attempting to bring some sort of causal explanation to the upholding of these attitudes. The reader must be directed to the actual volume for further study of this, but one can quote one example to indicate the type of explanation offered. Thus in the case of the "Right" attitudes there is a loyalty to a leader, a single father-figure, whereas in the "left" there is loyalty to the group. Flugel now links this up with the theoretical writings of Freud as portrayed in the more social psychological and anthropological books. What is attempted as an explanation for the "right" and "left" views depends upon the theory that leaders are as it were recapitulations of one's experiences with one's own father. On the one hand there is a feeling of respect, love and homage towards the father, on the other there is a tendency towards rebellion, feelings of envy and hatred. When these early sentiments are reproduced in later life toward other people, there is a tendency for them to be attached to definite social attitudes. "The attitude of the 'right' thus corresponds to the universal human tendency to loyalty towards parents and parent substitutes, that of the left represents the no less ubiquitous conspiracy of the young against the old. Since

[29] Flugel, J. C. *Man, Morals and Society*. Pelican Books 1955.

both attitudes are inevitable, it is not surprising that parties crystallise around them, calling to their banner those in whom one or other attitude happens to preponderate, and that, just as revolution follows tyranny, so counter-revolution follows revolution."

When talking of a conservative or a radical pattern, we are talking at a relatively "high" level of explanation. Once again it must be reminded that we do not "see" an attitude. It might then be legitimately asked by a practising caseworker, of what use is all this to me? The answer lies in the fact that we have already noted, namely that opinions are seldom isolated from one another. So that an individual conviction regarding discipline in a client's family might be expected to go with fairly strong views about religious practice and so on. It must be said, of course, that such factors as conservatism-radicalism are inferred generalisations from a great number of cases, and therefore the particular case that one meets may not be easily deduced from these. Nevertheless if one is able, by virtue of a scientific explanation, to bridge an otherwise isolated number of facts under one head, and to provide some measure of prediction, there is a considerable practical advancement made.

Racial Attitude and Social Work. With regard to racial attitude, we might refer to its relevance in social work. On the purely personal level it is clear that differences in colour (to take this aspect of race) must make a difference in a worker-client relationship. This may shift from country to country and from area to area, according to the degree of the views held regarding this. But to take an American study,[30] it was found that the attitude most likely to be shown in Negro clients in a northern child guidance clinic was that of open hostility, and until the question of colour was tactfully brought out into the open, there remained this feeling of hostility. The reaction may be different in other places; it is sufficient to indicate that racial attitude must be taken into account.

CHANGE

Having discussed the formation and maintenance of both habits

[30] Verin, O. "Racial attitudes of Negro Clients". *Smith College Studies in Social Work* 1945, *16*, τ.

and attitudes, there remains the pertinent enquiry as to the possibility of altering them. Observation of historical development shows us that changes have occurred in societies, albeit in some cases slowly and with difficulty. Nevertheless some sort of progress has been made. Common observation of individuals again indicates that they are capable of altering their views and conduct, although again with difficulty. In view of the obvious difficulties that people have in changing their customary ways, one might posit the question whether there is something inherently conservative in Nature. The answer to this lies in heredity and to the persistence of an established structure. Sir Charles Sherrington[31] in an interesting passage exemplifies the "toryism" of Nature with respect to the penguin. "On the Antarctic ice the penguin, since first it was a penguin, can never have seen a tree. It cannot fly. The wing is dwarfed to a little paddle. Under it the head cannot possibly be tucked away, the wing is far too small. Yet faithful to the habit of forbears thousands of years before, the penguin when it composes itself to sleep turns its head and puts the tip of the beak, it can no more, under its midget wing." Human beings may be somewhat unlike penguins in other respects, but with respect to customs and traditions there is a similar harking back to the past, although not in the strict biological sense in the example of the penguin. One need not invoke more than a lifetime; everyday life presents plenty of examples to show us that to go against the early socialising and educative influences of childhood is to go against the grain. The force of habit may not be of a mechanical nature, yet it is nevertheless very strong.

We shall therefore be taking up the subject of change as synonymous with alteration and not with development, about which the last section was partly concerned. In the present section we shall be drawing the threads of habits and attitudes together to a common aim, namely that of altering them. In order to discuss the various methods and involved difficulties of doing this, it is first of all necessary to discuss the resistance to change. There is no need to labour the point that indirectly effecting change is precisely what the social worker is doing. He may not be saying explicitly that the client has to do this instead of that, or not do this instead of that, or even trying to change a point of view

[31] Sherrington, C. S. *Man on his Nature*. Cambridge 1940.

directly. Yet there is no doubt that the idea of change—of altering an undesirable reaction, or an individually harmful or incomplete outlook—is fundamentally there. And even if it is not explicitly there in the social worker's practical repertoire, the idea of the possibility of altering the customary state of affairs must enter into the interpersonal relationships. Certainly a study of the factors involving the resistance to change and the difficulties in altering any given piece of behaviour is one that must contain practical suggestions. Individuals differ, and so do circumstances, yet there is sufficient common ground to be able to select the chief features on the subject which we are now discussing.

RESISTANCE TO CHANGE

The fact that people do show sometimes an overwhelming resistance to some alteration in their way of life or way of looking at things is too well known to amplify by examples. What is pertinent is to inspect some of the major forces inducing the resistance.

Age. It might be asked at the outset, proceeding from common observation, how much has age to do with the clinging to old and familiar attitudes? What experimental evidence there is on this point accords with common belief, namely that the older a person is, the more difficult it is to change his viewpoint. Thus in one investigation, Marple[32] attempted to change the attitudes on certain controversial problems of 900 people, divided into thirds of high-school students, the average age of whom was eighteen; college students, average age twenty-two; and adults, average age thirty-nine. The degree of change of attitudes, from most to least, was in the order presented above, thus indicating that age has much to do with change of attitude. On the other hand it is clear that some people, even at an advanced age, are capable of change, and one would like to know more about individual differences, the circumstances in which change is introduced, the particular nature of the change, and so on. In other words, although the common belief that as one gets on in years one is less open to new things may be true, it leaves out, as a generalisation, some of the interesting exceptions to this, which may prove to be more important than the rule itself.

[32] Marple, C. H. "The comparative susceptibility of three age levels to the suggestion of group versus expert opinion". *J. Soc. Psychol.* 1933, *4*, 176.

Sources of Resistance. Resistance may have very different sources, as Kelly and Volkart have noted.[33] Resistance to change may spring from an inner conviction that one is right, or a person may fear to change because of the expectation of punishment if he wanders away from the accepted state of affairs. The first distinction refers to people who are bound up with their attitudes, "ego-involved" as it is put. Newcomb[34] has put the case neatly: "When a person perceives an influence as a force opposed to some attitude of his which is ego-involved, he is apt to counter that force with other forces of supporting nature. He becomes motivated not only toward the object about which he has an attitude . . . but also toward the defense of his own self. Under such conditions his attitudes are maintained or even intensified in spite of influences which threaten to change his attitudes". Therefore an elderly person who has cherished feelings towards the objects in her room, the knick-knacks and furniture which she has had for years, is apt to present a barrage of defences when these things are threatened. Certainly ego-involved attitudes are those in which there is the most resistance to alteration. Why should this be so? It is because it is not *just* an attitude that is being threatened, it is in fact the person himself, or part of him. The most obvious examples on this score come from the protocols of patients undergoing psychotherapy, though it is also evident if one listens to debates or discussions of theories, in which the protagonists and antagonists have given much of their years and energy to the matters discussed.

The other type of failure to change is represented in the tendency not to deviate from the stock beliefs of one's group or society. "Punishment" in such a case may vary from social sanctions (such as being sent to Coventry) to mere ostracisation, and in these instances it may be the *expected* consequences rather than the actual consequences that are the operative influences.

Both these sources are regarded from the point of view of the individual being aware of his own attitudes which he does not want to give up, but it is clear from psycho-analytic and similar findings that the most intransigent attitudes are those which are

[33] Kelley, H. H. and Volkart, E. H. "The resistance to change of group-anchored attitudes". *Amer. Sociological Review.* 1952, *17*, 453.
[34] Newcomb, T. M. *Social Psychology.*

only partly conscious. Then a person may resist any innovation which threatens his feeling of security without being altogether certain as to why he has this further feeling of threatening loss. Attitudes which are only partly conscious are held on to with all the more force. In extreme cases it leads to maladjustment.

Perception of change. A point which requires a little further amplification is the fact that to be a threat, an undesirable change must be *perceived* as such. To take a modern example: automatic machines have been in operation for some time, there have been innumerable articles about them in the popular press, even articles which stressed the possibility of redundancy resulting from the universal use of them. Yet it is only comparatively recently that the British worker has perceived them as a threat (rightly or wrongly, it is of no consequence in the present argument). Resistance to the use of automatic machines then comes as a direct result of perceiving their consequences; without the perception they are not regarded in any threatening light, even with interest perhaps. A rider to this might consist in the idea that the most successful innovations have been those that have taken place without people being aware of their possibilities. Then, too, there is always the fact that anticipated innovations are tinged with overtones that are different to the situation when the innovation comes about. All kinds of technological devices have been regarded, in their inception, in suspicious light. Railways, radio, television—all these have been labelled in their origins as being detrimental to the public interest, to health and so on. And whatever may be the truth of these dismal prophecies, the fact remains that it does not take very long before there is a complete reversal of attitude, or if not a reversal there is an indifference which reflects the lowering of resistance.

All this discussion is merely preparatory to an analysis of some of the ways in which habits and attitudes can best be altered without spoiling something in the process. It is apparent that resistance plays a useful role. If everybody had what the advertisements for Pelmanism call a "grass-hopper mind", then society would be in a chaotic state. Resistance plays a necessary stabilising part in the great machinery of society. At the same time a study of the history of ideas shows only too clearly that this can be overdone, with the frequent result that a useful invention is held up.

It is also apparent that resistance mainly comes from those who are most proficient in their special disciplines. A perusal of the attitude of the Royal Society in the past sometimes make depressing reading. Nevertheless it is difficult to tell how much of this type of attitude may be necessary.

ALTERATION OF HABITS

We have previously discussed some of the ways in which habits are formed and sustained. Now when it comes to *changing* a habitual response, it depends very much upon what sort of habit it is as regards the path of transformation we take. Clearly we do not take the same measures for emotional habits as we do for manual ones. Yet basic to all the types there are principles which are common ground. It may be largely axiomatic, though still necessary to stress, that motivation must play the initial part. An alteration of any single habitual sequence is not liable to be successful unless it is really desired, and desired not in any sense of being a pious wish but a definite aim backed up with appropriate measures. The aim, though, is not enough. Exclusive attachment to the aim to be achieved does not result in successful liberation from the undesired habit. There has to be, as has been said, appropriate measures. And the word "appropriate" may be emphasised because there are always inappropriate measures. Alongside the need for change, and somewhat integrated with it, is the awareness of the habit that is to be altered. There is an entire group of gestural and postural habits that is performed daily without any awareness whatever. It is not until a member of this group gives trouble in some way or another that we pay heed to it. A person may be an inveterate nail-biter, for example, without being aware of the fact that he is continually bringing his hands up to his mouth. He may catch himself in the act, but the sequence of the movements prior to this escapes him entirely. Therefore it is not unreasonable to suppose that part of the necessary steps in the alteration of a habit such as this consists in being aware of what one is actually doing when it is performed. This is not the whole story. There is the factor of familiarity to be considered. A familiar way of doing something brings with it a security; to deviate from the usual track brings with it a feeling of insecurity. In this there are large individual differences. Some people seem not to mind this at all and stray willingly from a fixed line of existence. Others are exactly the reverse; the quotidian repetition of events is associated with a feeling of liking for the usual and known; to depart from this is in the nature of a rupture.

Conditioned Reflex Therapy. One method of arousing awareness of bodily actions is contained in the application of conditioned response theory to bed-wetting.[35] The child who persistently wets his bed at night long after the age when a normal control of the bladder has matured, does so because he is not aware of the pressure on the bladder. If he can be made aware of this, by some mechanical means, then he stands a chance of relieving himself before the act takes place. Accordingly a contrivance has been designed whereby an electrical circuit attached with a bell is closed when urination takes place. The whole machinery consists of a specially designed pad, screened on either side with metal, and usable as a mattress, which only acts as an electrical circuit when it is wet. The ringing of the bell wakes up the child, and he goes to the lavatory. If this is used repeatedly there comes a time when the child becomes aware of the distension of his bladder, and thus able to break the habit. A psycho-analyst would probably object in principle to this method on the grounds that there was an underlying reason, such as a lack of interest by the father, which had not been dealt with by this method of eradication, and therefore it was only a symptom that had been dismissed and not the cause. This is quite possible of course, and the example is not presented as an argument against psycho-analytic doctrine. It is only given to.indicate how a particularly annoying habit can be dealt with by means of conditioning procedure. In the same way application of negative conditioning—the learning of how *not* to respond to a stimulus—can be brought about. Assuming that reinforcement is basic to conditioning, one can see how the old method of applying mustard to the fingers of the nail-biter works. The original habit is kept up because the habit is satisfactory to the offender. The conditioning is "de-conditioned" by changing the satisfying effect. The effect becomes in fact unpleasurable and the particular habit is dropped because the sustaining factor of satisfaction has been taken away from it.

Awareness can also be brought about by a deliberate inculcation

[35] Mowrer, O. H. *Learning Theory and Personality Dynamics.* Ronald 1950.

of the undesirable response. Dunlap[36] gives the example of a person persistently writing "hte" on the typewriter. To overcome this particular misspelling the writer is made to deliberately type out the incorrect spelling many, many times. In this way the actions of the fingers is brought home to the person and he thenceforth avoids this habit.

Stages in habit-breaking. Dunlap also considers the steps necessary in the breakdown of emotional habitual responses, such as bad temper, irritability, apathy and timidity. He recognises that there is involved four stages. At the outset the patient must be clearly comprehensive of the nature of his difficulties in the sense that he is aware of the inadequacy of the habit, and the effects of it in his life. The second step consists of forming or accepting "the proper ideals, conceiving as clearly as possible of the results which will accrue from the elimination of the habits". In other words he must be aware of the harm of the particular habit he has and must realise, inversely, what benefits he will receive from its elimination. This of course is hardly sufficient, and the third step is a proper motivation to discard the old and strive in the direction of the new. Yet even this is still insufficient, and the final step lies in engaging "seriously and persistently in the practice which is outlined for him as a means to the desired end." As addenda to this one should notice that there may be quite a gap between stages three and four, which in itself could consist of a number of intermediary steps. Also there is the fact that a person may as it were fool himself that he desires a habit to be changed. It is one thing to wish strongly the night before that one will arise early, contrary to the usual practice of lazing in bed. It is quite another thing when the alarm bell rings at six or seven. It is quite a conceivable fact that the motivation dies out as a direct result of a taste of the measures that are required in order to carry out the original motive. Transforming habitual behaviour is no light matter and requires a constant interplay of desire and practice in order for it to be completely successful.

ALTERATION OF ATTITUDES.

It is not so difficult to experimentally reproduce situations in which a number of subjects are exposed to attempts to alter their

[36] Dunlap, K. *Habits: Their Making and Unmaking.* Liveright 1932.

outlook on various matters, and there have been in fact a number of studies which have done this. These studies have been carried out with the intention to discover just what are the main factors which induce change, and which are the factors which prohibit it. If one takes such a matter as attitudes towards Negroes as a starting point, one might speculate as to the ways an unfavourable attitude may be overcome. There are, in the main, two possible methods. One may hear a talk about Negroes, or read about them or something very similar, on the one hand; on the other hand one can actually meet Negroes, talk with them and have dinner with them. One may wonder which of these two methods would be more successful in inducing a favourable reaction. Experimental studies confirm that both methods *do* help to assist a favourable attitude, but the first method only slightly.[37] For example students who had undergone a course of lectures on Immigration and Race Problems showed that their attitudes towards Negroes were improved, as compared with a comparable set of students who had not taken this course. The other method, also performed at an American University, in which the students were taken around Harlem and met and ate with Negroes, showed a large yield in the favourable direction. Moreover when these students were tested nearly a year after the tour over a half of the students had still kept their altered viewpoint about Negroes. This, of course, is an encouraging indication and leads to the conclusion that all that is required for alteration of racial prejudice is sufficient degree of familiarity. Yet there is more to it than this. It must be remembered that even in this study the tour was conducted with the *imprimatur* of the university. That is to say for the students there was an implicit understanding that their authority countenanced and encouraged familiarity with Negroes. In a prevailing atmosphere in which this may be the reverse, it is doubtful whether *mere* familiarity is sufficient.

Change of Group-anchored attitudes. A knowledge of the habitat of other people, and especially meeting them on equal terms, then, is partly successful in producing a change of heart. Very often this is the whole story. To have been brought up in the belief that Jews are dishonest and then to come across a few that clearly are not,

[37] See the studies by Smith, M. and Smith, F. T. in Krech and Crutchfield: *Theory and Problems of Social Psychology*. Chapter VI.

has enough demanding force to do away with the original attitude. Yet there are cases in which there is more complexity than
this. We have already seen that resistance to change is made all
the harder when the group to which one belongs is conservative
in this direction. What was made clear in the study by Kelly and
Volkart to which we referred earlier, was that one of the main
factors was the extent to which somebody valued their own membership in the group. Kelly and Volkart tested the attitudes of
Boy Scouts regarding camping and woodcraft activities. (These
particular boys being of urban origin.) They were tested about
these activities both before and after listening to a speech in which
there was criticism of the Scouts' emphasis on these activities, and
in which there was recommended substitution of various city
activities. The experiment had a further complication in that this
same speech was performed under private conditions for some of
the Scouts and under public conditions for others. In addition a
Scout's valuation of his membership in the group was ascertained
from a questionnaire. Now it was thought that the extent to
which a Scout would be influenced by the speech would be inversely related to how highly he thought of his membership in
the group. That is to say, if he thought of himself as being very
high in the Scout group, the less likely it would be that he would
be affected by the criticism. And especially would this be so if the
listening was done under public conditions. This hypothesis is
related as the authors note "to the theory and literature dealing
with conformity to group norms, publicness of attitude expression,
and internalisation of social norms." It is not surprising to find
that the results confirmed the assumption. The more identified
one is with a group—and this becomes more intense the higher
up one is in it—the more likely is it that the values of the group
are accepted, and the more likely is it that an effort to effect a
change in attitude is resisted. And especially if others in the group
would be likely to be aware of a change in one's attitude. If there
is to be a radical change it is expected that there also must be a
change in social attitudes or personality structure or both.

Group decision and discussion. In this study there is revealed the
important part which communication plays between the members
of a group acting as a group. This last point has been made quite
clear by all those experiments made during the last war on the

effectiveness of propaganda for various eatables between lectures by authorities and taking a group decision.[38] All results indicated that the latter method was the more successful. In these experiments "resistance to change" had reference to the failure of American housewives to buy such eatables as beef hearts, sweetbreads and kidneys. Although special lectures were given on the importance of nutrition for the war effort and the vitamin value of these foodstuffs was emphasised, there was no great alteration in their sale. A *discussion* by a group of housewives about these foods and the whole problem of food and the war, produced quite a different effect. Group participation and discussion therefore is an important point, and the effect of these can be seen in quite another field, namely in factory work. Here a study by Coch and French[39] makes it quite apparent that group meetings and participation by the group in planning of changes can be of assistance in the overcoming of resistance to them.

Group decision and participation is possibly only successful when there is a strong group feeling. This may seem tautologous, but one can talk of close-knit and loose groups, and it is with the first that there appears success. Cartwright[40] makes this his first principle in considering the group as a medium of change. ". . . those people who are to be changed and those who are to exert influence for change must have a strong sense of belonging to the same group." The lesson to be learned from all this is plain: in order to introduce a novelty, against which there may be some resistance, one way of getting it across is to make clear to those who are concerned that the issue is with them and that their participation and opinion is required. At any rate the evidence shows that nothing is lost by this device.

[38] See Lewin, K. "Group decision and social change". In Newcomb and Hartley *Readings in Social Psychology*.

[39] Coch, L. and French, J. R. P. Jnr. "Overcoming resistance to change". *Hum. Rel.* 1948, *1*, 512.

[40] Cartwright, D. "Achieving change in people: Some applications of Group Dynamics Theory". *Hum. Rel.* 1951, *4*, 381.

IV

PERCEPTION

THE German psychologist Koffka once introduced the study of perception by stating the question: "Why do things look as they do?", a question which might be supplemented by further enquiries of "Why do people appear as they are?" and "Do other people see me as I see myself?" The subject of perception can be studied from different viewpoints; answers to the first question will be discussed in the first two sections of this Chapter, answers to the second and third questions, in the last two sections.

THE PROCESS OF PERCEPTION

Perhaps the most astonishing fact about our perception of things and people, is that they appear to be not a mass of impressions but assume a recognisable organisation. An apple does not appear to us as a combination of complex sensations of shape and colour; it merely is—an apple. Sensation is aroused by the interaction of our sense organs with energy in the form of electromagnetic waves outside of us. Seeing, for example, is the result of waves reaching the photosensitive layer of the eye which is called the retina. Hearing is the result of waves stimulating the eardrums. From the retina and the eardrums electrical impulses are transmitted along the nerve fibres to areas in the brain (the cerebral cortex: see Chapter VI) which receive these impulses. When this process is completed, we say "I see the apple" and "I hear the bell". If we regard perception solely from this point of view of the transmission of sensations we might conclude that "so far as the receptor areas of the cortex were concerned, the external environment would be supposed to consist of a mass of sight, sound, taste, smell, touch, pain, heat and cold, pressure, joint and muscle sensations, each differentiated more or less

accurately in intensity, extensity, localisation, and duration; and
also in certain qualities such as colour, pitch, etc., which were
peculiar to the type of sense organ stimulated".[1]

Wholeness. What we perceive however is not just an assortment of
different sensations but a distinct meaningful object. The classical
atomistic school of thought had supposed that our perceptions
were built up from our sensations rather like a brick wall is made.
Just prior to the beginning of the first world war three German
psychologists, namely Max Wertheimer, Kurt Koffka and Wolf-
gang Köhler, started the Gestalt line of thought which by a
wealth of clear-cut experimentation, demonstrated that our perceptual experience cannot be described in terms of elements but
in terms of wholes, and proceeded to demonstrate the principles
of organisation involved in the perception of wholeness. As such
the emphasis is not on sensations but on the *sensory field*, not on
individual elements but on the *"configuration"* of them. The Gestalt
school had repercussions not only in the field of perception but
also in learning and thinking and many other fields. We need only
note here the application to perception. The meaning of this line
of thought is exemplified by the problem originally raised by von
Ehrenfels: how is it that if I play a familiar tune in a different key,
that tune is still recognisable? Obviously there must be something
more than the notes making up that tune? In other words the
arrangement of the notes is a factor that must be taken into account.
Now it is this form quality in all our perceptions to which the
Gestalt school called attention and which gave rise to the catch-
phrase of the movement that the whole is more than the sum of its
parts. This was not by any means the only contribution made by
the Gestalt writers to perceptual study, but it forms the cornerstone of their ideas. As an example to portray their ideas the
"phi-phenomenon" can be cited. This effect is basically brought
out by briefly showing a fixed line of light followed after a very
short time interval by another fixed line. If the arrangements of the
lines in distance and temporal interval from one another are
right, there is formed the illusion of movement. That is to say
the first line will appear to move in the direction of the second
line of light. Neon advertisement signs as of a man pouring out
whisky are based on the same principle—one does not see a line

[1] Vernon, M. D. *A Further Study of Visual Perception.* Cambridge 1952.

of lights but one gains a whole impression. From the theoretical point of view it can be seen that the appearance of movement could not be predicted by the mere summation of its parts, the two lines in this case. There is added a third factor namely the particular configuration of the two lines which resulted in the illusion of movement.

Gestalt psychology is not the only representative theory in the study of perception,[2] and there is no doubt that by an emphasis on the present organisational properties, the effect of past experience has been overlooked. It has proved amazingly fruitful, though, and many concepts in continual use in psychology, such as "field", owe their prominence to the Gestalt approach.

Perceptual Constancy. Not only do we attribute "wholeness" to the world of objects and people, we also have the tendency to form a certain stability to them. Objects do not appear to fluctuate under differing conditions of illumination and distance. We still see a penny as a circle even in conditions when the image of the penny describes an ellipse on the retina. A man in the near distance still appears to be the same height as he is when near to us. A piece of coal appears to be black even in bright sunlight. Examples could be multiplied; the phenomenon is known for shape, size, brightness and colour, within limits. It points to the fact that it is biologically important for the organism that the environment about it holds to some constancy. The world would become an impossible place if it was seen as a continually changing kaleidoscope. Some regularity must be imposed.

As a matter of experimental fact it is known that for shape constancy, at any rate, there is a compromise between the "world as it is" and "the world as it is projected on to the retina". Thouless[3] found that if he asked a number of subjects to match a circular disc with several ellipses of differing ratio, the average result lay between the circular shape of the disc and the elliptical shape of the image on the eye. This tendency for the retinal shape to be distorted towards the direction of the object is called the phenomenal regression to the "real" object.

[2] For the present status of theories of Perception see Allport, F. H. *Theories of Perception and the Concept of Structure*. Wiley 1955.

[3] Thouless, R. H. "Phenomenal Regression to the Real Object. *Brit. J. Psychol.* 1931, *21*, 339 and *22*, 1.

There is considerable individual variations in the constancy phenomena, and at present there is no satisfactory theory regarding their operation.[4]

FUNCTIONAL ASPECTS

The distinction has been made between the "structural" determinants of perception on the one hand, and the "behavioural" determinants on the other.[5] By structural determinants is meant the effect on perception of the nature of the stimulus, the influence of the sense organs, nerve paths and the receiving areas of the brain, and also what we have already discussed in the last section. The behavioural determinants include the effects of past experience, and the systems of needs and values, which we will now proceed to summarise.

LEARNING

As Hilgard[6] has put it, it comes as quite a jolt to find out how easily the "copy" theory of perception can be exploded. The analogy between the eye and the camera, the ear and the microphone, and between the taste buds and chemical indicators seems very plausible. However, the real situation is not like this at all. There is not a passive registration. It is more like an active selective organisation. The most convincing demonstrations of this stem from the experiments carried out at the Hanover Institute. These demonstrations have made quite clear that our perceptions are built up from a whole group of similar occurrences, upon which we base a statistical presumption. They elaborate in more detail and with considerably more understanding the simple saying that a burnt child fears the fire. If we find by experience that a "reddish flickering thing" hurts us, and that a second

[4] But see Taylor, J. G. and Papert, S. "A theory of perceptual constancy". *Brit. J. Psychol.* 1956, 47, 216.
[5] See Chapter 13 of F. H. Allport's book (*op. cit.*). The distinction was made by Bruner and Postman.
[6] Hilgard, E. R. "The role of learning in perception". In Blake, R. R. and Ramsey, G. V. *Perception: An Approach to Personality*. Ronald 1951. This chapter quotes the demonstrations of the Hanover Institute. For the original see Ames, A. *Nature and Origin of Perceptions* (Preliminary laboratory manual). Hanover Institute 1949. The present author is indebted to the Blake and Ramsey volume for guidance to selection of material in this section.

similar phenomenon has the same effect, and still a third, we tend to presume that all such phenomena will result in our being hurt if we touch them. An example of one of these experiments is the case of playing cards displayed in a special apparatus which does not disclose the distance from the observer. Now a standard-sized playing card is seen at its correct distance, while an over-sized one appears closer than an under-sized card. This is understandable. But now the same procedure is done with oak leaves. There is of course no standard sized oak leaf. But as Hilgard points out in a description of these experiments, "The fact is that each person has his own standard-sized oak leaf. In the ambiguous situation he sees any oak leaf, whether large or small, according to his preconception as to how big a standard oak leaf is. Then he places it perceptually at a distance that fits this preconception."

This is only one example of the Ames demonstrations; there is a whole group of artificially constructed illusions which establish the same principle, and indicate how our phenomenal world is made up and how the organism contributes to its own perceptual field. The influence of the past, however, can be a double-edged tool. This is neatly seen in a little experiment performed by Adams[7] with artificial flowers. She displayed a pink rose, a red rose and a bunch of violets. The pink rose was perfumed with violet, the red rose with lily and the violets with lily. Despite this, most of the subjects reported that the perfume they smelled was the characteristic odour of the flower given to them, even though when they were tested with their eyes closed the scents were identified correctly.

The foregoing experiments go to show that our various perceptions are not bundled at random within us. Not only do we pay attention to what concerns us, we also have assumptions about what we shall see or hear or smell or feel. This is again obviously a pragmatic device without which we would find the incessant stimuli of the outside world a very confusing array.

Learning after Blindness. Not only are our perceptions built up in this fashion, but there is evidence to show that different modalities of sense combine to form a meaningful world. There are two

[7] Adams, G. K. "An experimental study of memory color and related phenomena". *Amer. J. Psychol.* 1923, *34*, 359.

groups of material on this point. The first[8] describes the way in which blind people, who have had their sight restored by surgical means, learn to see objects about which they have only had tactual and auditory information. The experience of these patients, on first using their visual sense, tells us that a person may realise that he is being stimulated visually yet is not able to identify the object in question.

Presented with a ball and a block, the patient can distinguish between them inasmuch as he could see that they were two different things, but he could not tell which was which visually, although he could tactually. Protocols of such patients indicate that colours are able to be identified easiest; motion, size and distance of objects next on the list of recognition; while identification of shapes may take months to master. It is an interesting fact that similar findings were found among chimpanzees who were artificially reared in complete darkness until they were sixteen months—at which age they mature.[9]

The Inverted Lens. The other grouping of material related to the inter-dependence of sense modalities and to the way the visual sense is learned, is represented by experiments with the inverted lens.[10] Normally, although the eye inverts the image of the observed world, we see the world as upright. A mechanical contrivance can reverse this so as to enable its wearer to view things upside down. People who have tried the experiment of employing an inverted lens for a period have discovered that although to begin with everything seems remarkably disorientated, a re-orientation takes place comparatively quickly. In other words the picture of the outside world resumes its usual upright framework. This has been known to take place in so short a time as one week. This is because a person can rely on his kinaesthetic and tactual information to merge with the unusual visual impressions. It bears out strongly the contention that we literally have to learn to see what in fact we do see.

[8] Reported by M. von Senden. Quoted in Hebb, D.O. *The Organisation of Behavior.* Wiley 1949.

[9] Riesen, A. H. "The development of visual perception in man and chimpanzees." *Science.* 1947, *106*, 107.

[10] The original experiments in this field were done by Stratton, G. M. "Some preliminary experiments on vision without inversion of the retinal image". *Psychol. Review.* 1896, *3*, 611.

MOTIVATIONAL ASPECTS

If the evidence relating to learning in perception has shaken the copy theory, the material relating to suggestion and "set" indicates that the perceptual apparatus is even more pliable still.

The role of suggestion is notorious and can be amusingly introduced with reference to an experiment made by Slosson[11] long ago. He opened a vial of distilled water before a chemistry class, informing the pupils that it contained a strong and powerful odour, and asked the class to put up their hands as soon as they smelled it. Whereupon a wave of hands rose up, starting from the front of the class and proceeding backwards. In fact the suggestion was so successful that some of the members of the class in the front seats complained that they felt ill and had to leave the room! Fink[12] also tells a story which further exemplifies the strength of suggestion. He had an asthmatic patient who complained that he was allergic to the smell of roses. When the patient saw a bowl of roses on the physician's desk he immediately had a paroxysm of coughing. The doctor then showed him that the flowers were made of paper. These two examples portray the effects of suggestion *in excelsis*, but the factor generally operates at a less obvious, and therefore more pernicious, level.

Set. "Set" refers to the condition in which the organism is in a temporary state of readiness to respond to a stumulus. With regard to a previous set, less extreme examples of the fact that we see what we expect to see is afforded by the use of ambiguous figures. These are drawings which have two alternative interpretations. Using one of this type of drawings, which characterised either a rabbit or a pirate among the contours of a countryside according to how one viewed the picture, Leeper[13] found that people reported seeing both figures in equal proportion. However if the subjects of the experiment had been previously given a similar drawing, but one in which either the rabbit or the pirate was delineated in a pronounced way, these same subjects on being subsequently shown the ambiguous picture, had some

[11] Slosson, E. E. "A lecture experiment in hallucinations". *Psychol. Review* 1899, *6*, 407.

[12] Fink, D. H. *Release from Nervous Tension.* Allen and Unwin, 1945.

[13] Leeper, R. "A study of a neglected portion of the field of learning—The development of Sensory Organisation". *J. Genet. Psychol.* 1935, *46*, 41.

difficulty in seeing the alternative interpretation—a difficulty which they had not in the first instance encountered.

All this material has much relevance to those engaged in activities where there is always a knowledge of an individual preparatory to the actual meeting, as for example in an interview. Generally the interviewer has already read some account of the person he is about to see, and inevitably on the strength of this previous history there is built up an expectation of what this person is like, perhaps even in a physical sense. Very often in this sort of situation we are agreeably surprised to find that the man or woman we had expected to see was not like that at all. Very often the reverse is equally true. But, as we shall again note when stereotypes are discussed, the important point is that the preperception should be amenable to change, should be plastic and not rigid, as it is difficult, if not impossible, to avoid any previous set.

Motivational Selectivity. The whole question of previous set is very much linked with motivational selectivity. It is indeed possible to influence a person's perception by introducing a system of rewards and punishments. Proshansky and Murphy[14] were able to induce their subjects to over-estimate lengths of lines by bringing in rewards when long lines were displayed and punishment when short lines were featured. While there does not seem enough empirical evidence to support the view that wish-fulfilment operates as a basic law in perception, this type of experimentation does lend credence to the statement that rewards and punishments "may play a significant role in the acquisition of perceptual response dispositions".[15]

Another feature of motivational selectivity is that to do with social pressures and cultural influences; this we shall reserve to the next section. What can be said in relation to motivation and perception, in short, is that the former introduces a further complexity. It is difficult, in any single case, to hazard the extent of this in relation to other deciding factors. In this, as in other matters touched upon here, it is enough to recognise that selectivity of this kind can be operative.

[14] Proshansky, H. and Murphy, G. "The effects of reward and punishment on Perception". *J. Psychol.* 1942, *13*, 295.

[15] The statement is by Postman, L. "The Experimental Analysis of motivational Factors in Perception". In *Current Theory and Research in Motivation*: A Symposium. Univ. of Nebraska Press 1953.

PERSONALITY

It should be apparent from a perusal of the last sub-section that perceiving can be exceedingly pliable. It is appropriate to round off the discussion by a consideration of some of the main individual differences.

There has been of recent years a growing body of literature on the relation between perception and personality, and at least three entire books on the subject. Here we will select one or two aspects in order to give an indication of the types of investigations involved. In some ways these have already been reflected in many of the studies quoted. Now attention will be paid to actual traits which bear witness to marked characteristics involved in the process of perceiving.

On the basis of experiments involving the manner in which people organised their impressions about the size of squares, Klein[16] found that there were two extremes. The actual experiment consisted in the judgement of the sizes of squares which were progressively altered in size. The extremes in reactions by the subjects were made up by those who kept constant pace with the systematic alteration, and by those who responded very slowly to change, who kept lagging behind and underestimating the sizes of the squares more and more. This distinction was tried out in other types of experiment and it was additionally confirmed that there were two definite kinds of perceivers—those who adapted themselves very well to change and those who clung to the old, or at least were reluctant to perceive things differently. Actually Klein designated three different dimensions of perceptual attitudes.

There was the dimension of Levelling versus Sharpening of differences (this applies to the above experiment with squares); there was the dimension of Tolerance versus Resistance to the unstable, that is adaptability to change or holding on to what is known; and there is thirdly the dimension which he called Physiognomic versus Literal, by which he refers to the fact that some people attribute to their percepts an emotional significance, while others are more inclined to call a spade a spade. These three dimensions of a general perceptual attitude are continua, so that any one person may lie in the middle of any single dimension, and

---

[16] Klein, G. S. "The Personal World through Perception". In Blake and Ramsey. *op. cit.*

they are not mutually exclusive, so that a person's position in them could be described by reference to all three.

Perception of the Unfamiliar. Of special interest for our purposes are the distinctions involved in rigidity of outlook versus plasticity, and the special feature which has come to be known as "Intolerance of Ambiguity". Together these characteristics make the point that there are strong individual differences in the way in which people react to the unfamiliar. Simple experiments as the one referred to above make the further point that there are many people who become "form bound", that is to say they find it difficult to give up the old habitual way of looking at things, and when they are thrust into a situation which is novel for them, they will cling to their habitually stable world. In other words there are people who prefer the "perceptual devil" they know to the one that they do not know. This is especially important to remember in those cases where a person has to leave his neighbourhood, or even his house, or where a radical change of occupation is imposed. The desire for stability and the clinging to the habitual is of course very prevalent in old age. If the series of experiments with artificially prepared perceptual situations can be generalised into conditions of life, it is useful for the social worker to know, as well as for others, that different people will react in characteristically different ways, to situations involving change, owing to the fact that there is a range of difficulty of re-adapting their *percepts*, and not simply in emotional and social ways of adjustment. Frenkel-Brunswick[17] has put this succinctly: "Results so far collected support the conjecture that, by and large, such tendencies as the quest for unqualified certainty, the rigid adherence to anything given—be this an authority or a stimulus—the inadequacy of reaction in terms of reality, and the like, operate in more than one area of personality. It can be demonstrated, further, that such specific forms of reaction as orientation towards concrete details (stimulus boundness) tend to occur again and again within an individual in contexts seemingly far removed from each other." Rigidity, therefore, is a factor to be encountered at all levels of personality, but it is also a factor embedded in a person's perception of his world and of himself.

[17] Frenkel-Brunswick, E. "Personality theory and perception". In Blake and Ramsey. *op. cit.*

SOCIAL PERCEPTION

Social Perception refers to the influence on individual perception of groups, classes, culture as a whole. It is not so much that there is a "working-class perception" or a perception peculiar to the Andaman Islands, say, which somehow exists apart from the perceptions of individual members of the working class or a solitary Andaman Islander, but that belonging to one or another of these groups makes a difference to the individual's perception. This may be a question of values—one selects perceptually those items which are in tune with the society one belongs to—or it may be a matter of learning. Learning, in its turn, is related to value, inasmuch as one only learns that which is relevant to the prevailing social climate, but they can be considered separately.

FIELD THEORY

The notions of "field theory" is particularly relevant to this subject. It is common knowledge what a field is in electricity and magnetism. A magnetic field is the region surrounding a magnet in which its influence can be detected. And in modern physics the concept of field has become an indispensable conceptual tool. Somewhat similarly the same concept has been valuable in psychology, and especially in social psychology, when important influences on people can be traced not only to their own motives, perceptions and personalities, but to the events which are happening around them. If one can imagine, in a naive simple way, a social belief acting as a magnet, then the people surrounding the magnet come under its zone of influence. The simile cannot carry us very far because of the fact that generally the "psychological" magnet is invisible, but the concept of the field enables us to carry explanation a step further than by just considering the manifest situation. In other words as Lippitt[18] once put it, this field approach enables us to study "the individual psychology of the group member and the collective behavior of the group regarded as a dynamic unity." By means of this concept there is achieved at one stroke a linkage of individual and social perception, and the two are related to form one dynamic whole. This is more than social factors just influencing an individual's perception; the two

[18] Lippitt, R. "Field theory and experiment in social psychology: autocratic and democratic group atmospheres". *Amer. J. Sociol.* 1939, 45, 26.

are regarded as extending over the same space and time in an integral manner.

Although we shall not attempt to translate the findings and speculations described in the rest of this section to field theory, it should be remembered that the latter is most relevant to the type of facts to which we shall be paying attention. "Cultural" and "social" fields of influence are no less important than the particular events which are enclosed in them.

GROUP INFLUENCE

Perhaps the best examples of group influence are the classic experiments performed by Sherif[19] on the autokinetic effect. This is an illusion, well known to old astronomers, of a point of light, if observed continuously in darkness, appearing to move. Sherif made use of this effect to study the impact of suggestion and group situation on perception. He investigated subjects, who were asked to judge the extent to which they thought the light had moved by pressing a telegraph key, under two conditions: when they were alone and when they were with others doing the same thing, that is to say as a member of a group. Subjects were either introduced to the group experiment first, and then went on to perform the judgement individually; or the reverse, they evaluated singly the apparent movement of the light first, and then proceeded to the group performance. In order to bring out the essential feature of this study it must be emphasised that here was a situation in which there was no possible external means of comparison in judging the movement of the light. In other terms the situation was highly "unstructured" and unstable. In view of the fact that each subject made one hundred judgements it might be thought that the net result of the judgements taken as a whole would be a scattered series of estimations. It was patently clear from the results, however, that the very reverse was the case. It was apparent that each individual subject had made for himself a scale and established within that range a standard. The standard or norm was different from individual to individual (when he was alone) but each had made a reference point for himself. Once established this would persist, as was noted when the experiment was continued on subsequent days. This alone is of interest, but

[19] Sherif, M. "A study of some social factors in perception". *Arch. Psychol.* 1935, No. 187.

we will postpone Sherif's conclusions until the group experiments have been described. In these the judgement of the extent to which the subjects imagined the light to have moved was spoken out aloud (so that all the members of the group heard it). Now in the case of those people who had come from a previous encounter with the light on their own, it was found that all the individual ranges and standards tended to converge to a common one. This "group effect" was noted too in the case of those who began *with* the group and in fact was stronger than the other way round. When the members subsequently split up into their solitary performances, the "group norm" was carried over into their single estimations. For the conclusions of this study we can best turn to its originator: "The experiments, then, constitute a study of the formation of a norm in a simple laboratory situation. They show in a simple way the basic psychological process involved in the establishment of social norms. They are an extension into the social field of a general psychological phenomenon that we find in perception and in many other psychological fields, namely, that our experience is organised around or modified by frames of reference, which are factors in any given stimulus situation."

Frames of Reference. The term "frames of reference" requires a special explanation. Everybody is familiar with the lines of longitude and latitude as drawn on a map in an atlas. Some point, say, in the middle of the Atlantic Ocean can be given an exact location by means of referring to these two lines. These have no absolute quality about them, they are simply relational to an agreed standard, which for longitude is Greenwich and for latitude is the equator. We might very well have designed them differently and chosen the South Pole as the standard for latitude, in which case practically everything else on the map would have been termed so many degrees north. When we come to standards of experience and behaviour there is the same procedure, only far less accurately defined. Judgements of experience or behaviour are seldom made in a psychological vacuum. They are made with reference, explicitly or implicitly, to a certain scheme of beliefs. These may change with experience, they may be prone to an easy usurpation by a different frame of reference, they may on the other hand persist through thick and thin, but they nevertheless are there. It is a characteristic of human mentality. Possibly the only exceptions to this are with extremely dissociated persons who are mentally ill. The results of Sherif's investigations indicate the interesting conclusion that it is an inevitable tendency in man to have a frame of reference. If this cannot be found in the external world, then it is developed. It is part of the human need for imposing order and structure on the incoming mass of impressions. Without some such ordering there would be a "blooming buzzing confusion". This applies not only to sense impressions, it also applies to the complicated levels of values and attitudes. Sherif's research shows us also that there can exist a group frame of reference which is paramount over an individual one.

SOCIAL CLASS

One way of defining social class is by reference to some object-ive criterion such as income or occupation. What is of relevance to social perception is the way in which people *regard* the things that count as "social class". The contribution of the social psy-chologist towards the definition of class consists in the way social class is defined by the *perceptions* of its members. One method of finding out this is by giving people a list of different occupational groups, such as doctors, farmers, waiters and many others, and asking them which they thought belonged to their own class. When this is done, as it was in an investigation of the American class structure by Centers,[20] it was found that the middle class was conceived, in terms of occupation, as either business or professional, a white-collar group; while the working-class was regarded as a manual group. Occupational status, however, was not the sole criterion: in response to the questions asked of each person as to whether he thinks it is important to know about a person's family, or how much money he has, or the type of education that he had, or the way in which he believes and feels about certain things, in deciding whether or not this person be-longed to the same class as himself, it was found that most people considered beliefs and attitudes to be the most operative factor. Education came next, followed by family and then money.

So much for the American scene. As regards this country, there has been an extensive investigation of how adolescents view

[20] Centers, R. "The American Class Structure: A Psychological Analysis". In Newcomb and Hartley: *Readings in Social Psychology.*

aspects of social class.[21] This research was undertaken to answer the questions, "To what extent do young adolescents view society in terms of adult frames of reference? Further, what are the relative influences of home and school in determining the boys' outlook?" The boys investigated came from different social and economic backgrounds, had different intelligences, and went to different types of secondary schools. The ages of the boys were from thirteen to fourteen. Compared with the way in which adults perceive social class, there was a striking similarity among the adolescents. A difference came in the regard of social classes other than the upper class (which both adults and adolescents characterised by the style of life); adolescents did not invoke the occupation criterion so much as adults. "There appears to be a tendency for adolescents to think of social classes more in terms of wealth or 'consumption patterns'." As a further step to enquire how adolescents perceived social class, it was asked of them what they considered to be the most important factors for evaluation. About sixty per cent of the sample tested considered personal effort, initiative, friendliness and ability to be most important, only fourteen per cent ascribed manners, dress and speech, and only ten per cent, education. The necessity of "good connections" was only attributed to by eight per cent. These were the over-all responses. It is interesting to note that middle-class boys in Modern schools were outstanding in attaching greater importance to speech and dress and manners generally, than to education. The authors explain this deviancy from the rest of the group by stating that the middle-class boy finds himself in the minority in the Modern School, and that because of this he is inclined to compensate by over-estimating the importance of appearance.

In answer to the second question—the relative influences of home and school in determining an outlook on social class—the solution lies in the fact that adolescents, like adults but more so, tend to rate their description of social class by the standard of their perceived position in it. In the case of these boys the prestige factor was that of the occupation of their father. However the influence of position in society was variable among the group. The views of the Modern School boys did not approximate so

[21] Himmelweit, H. T., Halsey, A. H. and Oppenheim, A. N. "The View of Adolescents on some aspects of the Social Class Structure". *Brit. J. Sociol.* 1952, *3*, 148.

closely to adult views as the Grammar School boys. The authors explained this difference as follows: "Apart from differences in the intellectual level of the pupils, these factors (that is the ones that make for the difference) include differences in the social class composition, academic status and tradition of the schools as well as in the range and status of occupations for which they prepare their pupils. Thus, the working-class boy in the Grammar School, by virtue of the education he receives, has already achieved a certain measure of upward mobility, whereas the middle-class boy in the Modern School has been to some extent downgraded and may find it difficult to take up a job which, in social standing, equals that of his father."

Finally, the authors' first conclusion should be emphasised, namely that although the term "social class" meant little to these adolescents, they had a good understanding of the present class system. Perceived class distinctions are doubtless a part of everybody's awareness in interacting with others, and may be as common as noticing that some people are well dressed and others are not. The perceptual clues may differ, some people placing more importance on dress and manners, others on education and others on factors more to do with personality. Whatever the emphasis, though, investigations have shown that "class distinctions" exists perceptually at any rate.

CULTURE

It is often written that sticking out the tongue signifies to the Chinese not rudeness, as it does in our own culture, but surprise, and it is only too easy to provide similar examples[22] and point out that different cultures have different modes of expression and communication, which may as in the above example, often be contradictory when one culture is compared to another. What is of further importance is that different cultures are differently perceptually motivated. What is of importance to notice in a highly technical urbanised existence is of little consequence in the Australian Bush.

Motivational selectivity, which we have previously discussed in the last section, might very well account for the differences in "cultural perception". One becomes so adhered to the perceptions particular to one's own culture that it sometimes comes as a

[22] See the section on "Non-Verbal Communication" in Chapter V.

shock that certain events are able to be regarded in quite another way, and as far as can be seen with equal justification. Take the example of measuring time. In our own culture we divide the day into hours, and our perception of passing time is more or less influenced by the clock. In many tribes, on the other hand, the day is divided according to other events.[23] In Hawaii there is a whole series of descriptions of the sun to demarcate time periods. This is how they describe the hours about dawn: "There comes a glimmer of colour on the mountains; the curtains of night are parted; the mountains light up; day breaks; the east blooms with yellow; it is broad daylight." As a contrast to this, terminology of periods of time in Madagascar are marked by such descriptions of events as "Cattle come home; the fowls come in; edge of rice-cooking pan obscure; people begin to cook rice; people eat rice; finished eating; everyone in bed." The different types of occupational interests and what is important for that community is reflected in the perception of time in the above example.

Other types of examples could be given. Cultural frames of reference are of importance to social workers particularly when immigrant groups are encountered. A newly arrived member from another country will not have had time to acclimatise himself to the outlook around him. His perceptions may still select those impressions which were of relevance to him in his old culture. On account of this he may very well feel lost or make mistakes of a perceptual nature. He may not understand why his new colleagues mistake certain of his intentions. All kinds of difficulties could arise from the unconscious employment of a different cultural frame of reference, and it may be part of the social worker's lot to help to clarify them.

STEREOTYPES

The term, originally coined by Lippmann, implies the development and usage, by pictures or models, of some category belonging to other people. Thus the racial category of "Jew" conjures up in some people an impression of somebody wily and avaricious. Shylock is the very epitome of a racial stereotype. The political stereotype of an anarchist still has overtones of a

[23] Sturt, M. *The Psychology of Time.* Kegan Paul 1925. Almost any event can be taken as a temporal index. Henry Koster in his *Travels in Brazil* 1817 noted that the inhabitants measured their age by the number of governors they had lived under.

wild man with bombs in his pocket. The essence of stereotyping is a labelling procedure. We carry round in our heads, so to speak, a picture of something or somebody which is only corrected if it is discovered to be hopelessly inaccurate. If we find what we expected all along then the stereotype is enriched. There is nothing essentially wrong about having stereotypes; in many ways they are useful devices. They select the universal feature in a number of varied elements. The drawback is encountered when this is applied too strongly in the social field, when the stereotype is held on to regardless of the evidence confronting it. This generally happens in the strongest form of prejudice when the individual literally refuses to perceive a fact contrary to his opinions, or looks for the minor points which support his stereotype and ignores the major points that would threaten it. Or again it can happen that although somebody recognises that his stereotype is inadequate, yet he clings on to it by making every example negating the stereotype an exception. Thus a colonial who has held strong anti-black views over a long period will regard each new coloured friend of her daughter as exception to the general rule of black people.

Experimental Examples. Experimental psychology contains plenty of information to amplify the whole conception of this subject. Rice[24] for example, displayed pictures to a number of students representing different personalities, including a steel magnate, a member of the U.S. Senate, a bootlegger, a financier, a Bolshevik, and others. The students were asked to report which type of individual belonged to which photograph. Most of the guesses were inaccurate, but the choices indicated that the selections were made on the popular conceptions of these types and not on any other grounds. Katz and Braly[25] used a different method of investigation. They gave a group of subjects a list of traits that were considered typical of ten racial groups, and the subjects of the experiment were asked to allocate these traits to the different groups. The results again showed the influence of the stereotype. Germans were described as industrious and methodical; Italians as musical

[24] Rice, S. A. *Quantitative Methods in Politics.* Knopf 1928.
[25] Katz, D. and Braly, K. "Racial Stereotypes of one hundred college students". *J. Abn. Soc. Psychol.* 1933–4, *28*, 280.

Perception

and imaginative: Negroes as lazy and superstitious. A somewhat similar investigation was followed in Hawaii[26]. There were groups of Japanese, Chinese, Koreans, Filipinos, Caucasian-Hawaiians, Chinese Hawaiians and Whites. These also were given a list of traits from which to select according to the type of characteristic which was thought typical of the others. All of the groups concurred in giving some leading idiosyncrasy to the remainder. There was unanimous agreement in describing the Japanese as polite, industrious, clean and neat. The Chinese were labelled industrious and shrewd; the Hawaiians as musical, easy-going and lazy. These two investigations, different in geography and in historical perspective, reflect remarkable unanimity. Stereotypes may alter according to changes of political climate; there is no reason to think that they will be dispensed with.

Evaluation of Stereotypes. What can be concluded from this feature in human beings? To begin with one should remember that the process of labelling is not peculiar to racial and political groups. It so happens that the term "stereotype" has become attached to these, but there is no logical necessity for it. We might very well have a stereotype of a table as being a surface with supporting legs. This is more or less accurate as it selects the universal feature of tables and ignores the differences that do exist. And if somebody had happened to have been brought up in the assumption that tables always had four legs, this would have been their stereotype, and a three-legged table would not have fitted into the notion. In this process there is a basic economy and simplicity. To quote Asch:[27] "Simplified impressions are a first step toward understanding the surroundings and toward establishing clear, meaningful views. Simplification often helps to see an entire situation clearly, to overcome the bewilderment and confusion of numerous details."

For anyone dealing with a number of people it is inevitable that stereotypes are formed. These may not be of the extreme type made known by literary works, by advertising or by comic strips. They are more of the nature of a mental synthesis and resemble

[26] Vinacke, W. E. "Stereotyping among national-racial groups in Hawaii: A study in Ethnocentrism. *J. Soc. Psychol.* 1949, *30*, 265.
[27] Asch, S. E. *Social Psychology*. Prentice-Hall. 1952.

more a character sketch than a parody. A health visitor may be forming a stereotype every time that she visits a certain neighbourhood. Mrs. S. who opens the door to her has the same sort of behaviour that Mrs. T. and Mrs. W. have in the houses adjoining. The health visitor may group them all together in one perceptual model, all with one chief characteristic, albeit with individual minor modifications. As has already been noticed, such a procedure is economical and necessary, to a point. The saving grace is the allowance of elasticity, otherwise stereotyping will forgo its labour-saving aspect and revert to a rigidity of outlook which blocks new impressions.

SELF PERCEPTION

The notion of what is meant by "self" has occupied the attention of philosophers and psychologists alike. For some it has been taken to mean the "knower", for others it has been the empirical "me". Some psychologists, like William James, have chosen organic sensations to be the basis of the self; others, like Köhler, have thought of the self as the central pivot of an abstract scheme, between up and down and between left and right. For our purposes we need not be concerned with the more philosophical aspects; we will merely deal with what Murphy describes as the individual as known to the individual.

It is often said that we fail to see ourselves as others see us; yet the truism, like many other truisms, fails to amplify what is most required, namely in what way we see ourselves, what type of mechanism is employed, the degree of truth or falsity about such self observations, and many other questions of a similar nature. It must be admitted that answers to these questions are not of such an exact nature as have been given in other enquiries; they only ascribe to indicate the *kind* of perceptions that various people in many different situations have made. The empirical fact is that the social worker continually comes up against this problem, and to some extent is required to see others as they see themselves. Furthermore there is the important fact that the way in which people see themselves at once influences and is influenced by their behaviour. The subject of self perception, then, is one that cannot be disregarded if one wishes to plumb deeper than the level of superficial behaviour.

SELF ESTEEM

For most people a certain amount of self esteem is a necessary piece of equipment for the daily transactions with other people. Too much of it or too little of it can lead to various forms of trouble. It is conditioned both by one's own opinion of oneself and by the consideration of what other people think. For many persons "whatever would people think" is a categorical imperative no less efficacious than the law, and as much a binding factor in self opinion as success at a job or failure at an examination. Comparison with others is another source of self esteem. In their textbook of Psychiatry Henderson and Gillespie[28] note that such comparison has two results. Either there is a feeling of satisfaction if the comparison is favourable, in which case the reactions flowing from this are adequate, or there is a feeling of failure, if the comparison is unfavourable, in which case there is again a twofold possibility. A person may try and do something about his deficiencies and correct the shortcomings of which he is aware, or else he may react in a negative way, "may shrink, become sensitive, self-effacing and dependent".

Success and Failure. Whether it is on account of one's own standards or because of other people's standards, judgements of success or failure is a factor that continually pursues a person's opinion of himself. G. W. Allport[29] points out that there are some people who prefer to make *certain* of success, and others who are characteristic in that they always try and bite off more than they can chew. This aspect of "level of aspiration" reflects the different types of self esteem. Allport goes on to state that younger children ordinarily prefer to repeat tasks in which they have already succeeded, while older children and adults prefer to work on tasks as yet uncompleted: "The older person battles against outer reality to retain his self esteem; the younger child in his world of pleasure prefers to hold on to his earlier and assured successes."

This aspect of self esteem can take many forms and can often be the source of self-recrimination against oneself. Take the instance of a mother of three children who regards herself as a failure, not because of material reasons as she admits that she

[28] Henderson, D. and Gillespie, R. D. *A Textbook of Psychiatry*. Oxford Med. Publ. 1950 ed.
[29] Allport, G. W. *Personality*. Constable 1937.

looks after them well in this way, but for other reasons. She thinks that she must have failed because they are so naughty; she compares them with other children and they do not seem alike. Here is an example of self esteem of one individual in the role of mother, judging herself to be lowered in her own regard because of some imaginary standard with other children. The craving for prestige in this case was associated with a fretful anxious personality. Sometimes, however, the craving for prestige can result in other ways. Karen Horney shows for example that it can take the form of a desire to humiliate others. Especially so in the case of those in whom self esteem has been wounded by humiliation in childhood. This process is most obviously seen in neurotics; it occurs in lesser degree in many where the deteriorating process has not gone so far.

Self Acceptance. Self esteem is bound up with self acceptance and the capacity to take criticism. Again these aspects show individual differences. There is the person who is extremely "touchy" on all matters reflecting his own conduct, while there are others who seem to be able to take any amount of criticism. Taylor and Combs[30] made a little experiment on this, taking as their starting point that people who were well adjusted would accept unflattering facts about themselves better than people who were less well adjusted. In the experiment children were asked to check a list of twenty statements, including such assertions as "I sometimes copy or cheat on school work", "I sometimes tell dirty stories", and "I sometimes am mean to animals", as being true of themselves. It was found, as predicted, that the better adjusted children checked significantly more of these self-damaging items than the others.

SELF DECEPTION

If self esteem can be regarded as a sentiment which enables us to keep our heads high in society, then self deception, from one point of view, can be considered as a type of mechanism which restores it when it is displaced. As Allport again remarks, it enables one to put off, for the time being, the admission of unpleasant truths until one is ready to receive them. This sort of

[30] Taylor, C. and Combs, A. W. "Self Acceptance and Adjustment". *J. Consulting Psychology.* 1952, *16*, 89.

deception, though, may very well continue throughout one's entire life, and of course the extreme forms of it can be found in the mental hospital.

Mechanisms of Deception. The mechanisms for deception are many and varied. First of all one may rationalise one's impulses. One can say to oneself, for example, after having failed at a particular task, "oh, well, I could have done that, only I didn't really try". The student who has done a bad examination and then excuses his results on the ground that he continually quoted authorities who were not known to the examiners represents another example. The inebriate who takes another sip "for his health" is a stock comic instance of such a mechanism. Then we may project on to others those qualities that we have in ourselves and of which we are ashamed; or sometimes the qualities that we think we ought to have, we find sadly lacking in other people. Katz and Allport[31] made an interesting study on cheating in students, in which the subjects were anonymous. Those who admitted cheating were the only ones who perceived cheating in others. The remainder of the subjects, who had not cheated themselves, did not report cheating in others. It can be seen from this that the first group tended to project their own wayward qualities on to those around them, although in this case admitting it in themselves, which is not always the case. Often projection is employed to avoid recriminations against oneself, and thus punishment is transferred from self to others. Guilt is projected, and we have the "scapegoat" theory of punishment. It can be said with some assurance that those people who are most verbose in judgement on the deficiencies and crimes of others, are those in whom an awareness of their own deficiencies and crimes is uppermost. Action against themselves is avoided by shelving the issue in pointing to other people.

These are two of the main mechanisms which are associated with deceiving oneself. Further mechanisms have been described by Frenkel-Brunswick,[32] in a study of which the aim was to compare the actual conduct of a group of students, as observed by

[31] Katz, D. and Allport, G. W. *Students' Attitudes.* Craftsmen Press 1931. See the Section "Psycho-Analytical Aspects" in Chapter VI for a further comment on projection.
[32] Frenkel-Brunswick, E. "Personality Theory and Perception". In Blake, R. R. and Ramsey, G. V. *Perception: An Approach to Personality.*

four independent judges, with the students' own statements about their conduct. The most striking mechanism which she found was what she called "distortion into the opposite". Thus the one student who was characterised by all the judges as insincere, declared himself to be sincere under all conditions. Distortion into the opposite is sometimes shown in those people who eagerly claim that they are the sort of person who would never indulge in gossip, and then proceed straightaway to do so. Exaggerated formulations, significant omissions, and minimising the importance of some events, were further mechanisms that were illuminated in the same study. "The lady doth protest too much" is often a sure sign that guilt feelings are being covered up in a welter of protestation. Similarly if in a mass of self observations the very thing that is expected to be of importance to the individual is omitted, we are entitled to have a shrewd suspicion that this is being left out on purpose, although the omission does not necessarily mean that it is conscious. "Minimising" is a little more difficult to see, and we may best turn to the author's own description. "Here a trait is seen by the subject in an unconcealed way but is minimised by his regarding it as not very strong or by his shifting the emphasis away from it by mentioning it relatively late in his self-characterisation. Thus in the case of one student all the judges had noted first of all in their list of traits that he was extremely social-minded, altruistic, and self-sacrificing. The student himself said, 'I try to help others if I can', but he put down this statement only after he had listed nine other traits in the description of himself."

Recognition of Oneself. Somewhat germane to the discussion of deception is the question of to what extent does a person recognise his own self. One of the most interesting researches on this was performed by Wolff,[33] who gave a number of subjects presentations of their own voice, profile, shape, hands and writing, together with other forms of expression, and asked them to compare these characteristics with similar characteristics belonging to other people. It is noteworthy to see that only sixteen per cent of the subjects recognised their own forms of expression in voice, and often it went to the extreme point of not recognising

[33] Wolff, W. "The experimental study of forms of expression". *Character and Personality*, 1933, 2, 168.

at all forms of expression as being their own. Yet in spite of this apparent limitation, the majority of those taking part in this investigation judged their own forms of expression more favourably than they did others and they were seldom neutral about their own characteristics. A similar experiment was performed later by Huntley[34] who found that in most cases the subject definitely preferred his own form of expression, although he was unaware that it was his own, and although when requested to point out his own in an assortment, failed to do so.

SELF IDEAL

The previous sections have tended to suggest that we have a picture of ourselves, a standard against which we are continually plotting our observations of our own thoughts and actions. It would be true to say that the more these two converge, the more adjusted becomes the individual. The less they converge, the less well adjusted. Horney has embodied this in her idea of the "idealised image",[35] which is having the defence of a faulty picture of one's virtues and assets. Another of her terms is "register" by which she means that one may know what is going on without being fully aware of it. If the ideal of the self is regarded as what the person would like to be but is not, then the manner in which these two approximate determines to a large degree a person's behaviour. Again it is similar to what has previously been discussed with the level of aspiration studies. If the carrot is placed too far ahead of the donkey the animal will very soon give up any hope of attaining it, and will perhaps resort to a dream carrot. Or if the vegetable, when taken, has a very different taste to what has been imagined, then again an imaginary carrot is regarded as more satisfactory.

Clearly, then, the unseen standard against which a man or woman places his or her potentialities is a very important factor in his or her make-up. We can cite as an example of this idealised image a rather sentimentally inclined foster mother who sees herself in a somewhat romantic light giving a home to a child whose real parents have been separated and the home broken up. After a while the make believe attitude which the foster mother has

[34] Huntley, C. W. "Judgements of self based upon records of expressive behavior". *J. Abn. Soc. Psychol.* 1940, *35*, 398.
[35] Horney, K. *Neurosis and Human Growth*. Routledge and Kegan Paul 1950

engendered dwindles under the powerful blow it receives from the behaviour of the child itself. The latter just does not come up to the expectation of the new mother; he becomes irritated by the false superficiality of the foster mother's behaviour and feels ill at ease. In turn, the self ideal pattern not developing as she has imagined, provokes in the foster mother a feeling of exasperation and dissatisfaction. The new alliance therefore becomes a failure, and is in fact a *mis*alliance.

Self or Ego ideal has repercussions far beyond the interior world of the individual who possesses it. Relatives and friends, interests and events will be incorporated in it also. Freud[36] connected it with the choice of a leader. He remarks that a leader will represent to the individual a clearer form of the latter's own qualities, together with greater force. The gap between ego and ego-ideal in most people not being too much separated, the leader will be an embodied self-ideal, a more marked picture of what the individual would like to become.

One should conclude that there is no particular detriment in having an ideal, even if it could be avoided. In fact it should be encouraged. The essential thing is that of the "distance" between what a person thinks he *ought* to be and what he thinks he *is*. Long ago William James[37] put this in the form of an equation where Self-esteem equals Success over Pretentions, about which he states that "the fraction may be increased as well by diminishing the denominator as by increasing the numerator. To give up pretentions is as blessed a relief as to get them gratified; and where disappointment is incessant and the struggle unending, this is what men will always do".

CHANGE OF SELF PERCEPTION

So far we have discussed how people observe themselves as if nothing further could be done about it; and in point of fact it is by no means an easy task for any fundamental change to take place. Sometimes, it is true, when adverse circumstances are mollified, the self-feeling associated with those circumstances clear up also. As, for example, a change of housing conditions may give to the occupant a rise in self esteem. Even a new Hoover may have an effect. But it is with the more important case that we

[36] Freud, S. *Group Psychology and the Analysis of the Ego.* Hogarth Press, 1922.
[37] James, W. *Principles of Psychology*, Vol. I. MacMillan, 1890.

are now concerned, where a man's awareness of himself is as much a part of him as a leg or an arm, and where a change in self-awareness is almost as much of an operation as an amputation, or at least a transplantation.

This is most noticeable in the type of person who comes for psychotherapy, and because the matter is accessible from this source, we shall quote material from here alone. It is also very relevant when medical after-care is considered. Take a man who has been in hospital for two years as a result of an accident, which has left him with the loss of the use of his legs. He has now got a job in a factory and is doing well. But what of the intervening period? What changes in his confidence had to be gained, the new self picture which was necessary to be built up in order for him to carry through a totally new life? Or, to take another aspect of life, consider the change in self esteem that has to be made by the young delinquent after his experience of remand home.

The position of people who want to undergo a change of self perception is analogous to the familiar picture of a person at the bottom of a mountain. He is unable to see the landscape from the position in which he is at the moment. In order for him to do this, somehow or other he has to ascend the mountain; and he can be assisted in this by another person who is able to see his plight more clearly than he can. Very often the mere pouring out of troubles to another person, and especially a sympathetic person, is sufficient to do this. In other cases it is necessary for an adviser to probe and spotlight the essential features involved. There can be no rigid rules laid down for this type of analysis. On the other hand there are certain precepts which are advisable to follow. Horney in her book *Self Analysis*[38] has discussed some of these. Frank and unreserved self-expression is the starting point. Without this there is doubt whether anything can be achieved, as otherwise there will always be a block on the outlet. At this point Horney makes two important conditions. The first is that the patient or client should attempt to express what he *really* feels and not what he thinks he is supposed to feel according to his own standards or to tradition generally. It is quite a commonplace in our own culture that one should not have feelings about hating one's parents for example. Horney insists that "he should at least be aware that there may be a wide and significant chasm between genuine

[38] Horney, K. *Self-Analysis*. Kegan Paul 1942.

feelings and feeling artificially adopted, and should sometimes ask himself—not while associating, but afterward—what he really feels about the matter." The other point is that the patient should try and express his feelings as much as he possibly can.

To effect a real change in an analysis of oneself, then, honesty must be a prerequisite. To give full expression to one's emotions and thoughts is something that not everybody can perform with equal ability. The problem of communication is one that must be transcended in addition to the problem of the analysis itself. Here is where the therapist, counsellor or advisor can assist by clarifying what the patient is merely seeing in an obscure way. He can often put matters in such a way that the patient is thus able to say, in effect, "yes, that is what I mean". To bear this out there is presented below excerpts from a recording of a woman who has undergone psychotherapy of the type known as the Client-centred approach, associated with the name of Carl Rogers.[39] At the twelfth interview this woman is saying: "I think what has happened to me is that . . . internally, emotionally, I don't know . . . I've sort of gone to pieces. That is, there have been breakdowns, not devastating ones, but it's almost as though you had a kind of physical structure, a piece of architecture, and there have been certain breakdowns, certain parts removed. And it's just not functioning well. And certainly the repair work hasn't set in yet, which. . . ." (Therapist): "You feel as though at the present time your structure is more impaired or less organised perhaps than it was when you came in, and the rebuilding of any newer type of structure to take its place hasn't really gotten under way." (Client): "That's right."

A later stage at which a reorganisation of the scattered and diffuse self perceptions takes place is very similar to the type of learning which has already been reviewed under the heading of insight. As the ape suddenly perceives that stick and banana are related to one another in his perceptual field, similarly the sort of person as the woman in the above example at once sees her difficulties in a new light. This may not be sudden; it may involve a long, tedious, and gradual process, and the stage at which insight is reached may not be so sudden and dramatic as the ape with the banana. The patient in the above quoted case also gave a neat

[39] Rogers, C. and Dymond, R. *Psychotherapy and Personality Change.* University of Chicago Press, 1954.

description of this latter period, when she says: "I keep having the thought occur to me that this whole process for me is kind of like examining pieces of a jigsaw puzzle. It seems to me I'm in the process now of examining the individual pieces which really don't seem to have much meaning." This may be considered to be at one of the primary stages. At a later period the pattern begins to emerge, the pieces form a meaningful whole, and the jigsaw is completed.

As was said before, this example of change of perception is borrowed from the clinical field because of the availability of data from this source, but the general process as outlined must happen in other situations in which there is an attempt to change the entire perception of oneself, whether it be *by* oneself or by others, or by a combination of both.

PERCEPTION OF OTHERS

Impressions of other people obviously depend on a number of conditions. There is the general situation at the time. A moment of marked emotional stress may make one perceive another person in a very different light from other, less intense, times. During war-time a soldier of the opposing nation may take the proportions of an evil character; a jovial policeman, to a young offender, assumes the likeness of a tyrant, and so on; further examples could easily be found. Impressions also depend upon one's general internal state at the time. A period of ill-health or run of bad luck may colour one's entire perceptions, and the world of others is placed into a category of either white or black accordingly. There is a poem by John Clare entitled "Written in Northampton County Asylum" in which he writes,

> ' Even those I loved the best
> Are strange — nay, stranger than the rest, '

which illustrates this negative aspect. Again, social suggestion may play a dominant role. The fairy story of the Emperor's New Clothes expresses the possibilities entailed in this in a very charming manner.

To bear in mind that any one person may be seen in very different lights by different people is something that is extremely necessary for the caseworker. *She* may see her client in a way that.

gives her no indication of the manner in which others see him. Indeed it is to be expected that her client would show a side of himself that he would not necessarily show to relatives or friends. The worker may sometimes wonder how it is that somebody else could possibly think this or that of her client. She may of course appreciate that other people have their own point of view and register their impressions accordingly; she may not actively realise that these same people may really *see* her client in a very different way.

In addition there is the factor of familiarity. We may have seen the same face so many times that we have built up an expected average of that face and cease to see anything new, and become mildly surprised after a lapse of time when there is a change. This again is a point which is of value for the worker to remember. She may see her client for a comparatively short period of time, six months say, yet the relatives and constant friends of the client are judging him from their particular temporal standpoint of some twenty to thirty years perhaps. Very often the reverse is also true; after a long period of time away one may expect one's friends to have changed in the meantime, especially if it is thought that oneself has, and then be rather put out to discover that they are just the same. There is a passage in one of Somerset Maugham's writings where he remarks that after a long period of travel abroad he returned to find that his friends were doing the same things, behaving in the same old fashion as they had when he had left them. The factor of time is one that is not easy to evaluate in this connection, although necessary to take into possible account.

FORMATION OF IMPRESSIONS

There is no doubt that we do not regard a person as a collection of isolated traits, of psychological bits and pieces. Asch[40] makes this point: "Although he possesses many tendencies, capacities, and interests, we form a view of *one* person, a view that embraces his entire being or as much of it as is accessible to us. We bring his many-sided, complex aspects into some definite relations. When we attempt to describe a person, we do more than enumerate the details of his actions. We specify his characteristics, but we do not stop at this point; we also bring his characteristics into relation. We contribute something to the grasp of a person; we

[40] Asch, S. E. *Social Psychology*.

organise the flow of observations in a somewhat ordered way." This Gestalt emphasis suggests that we form a composite picture of a personality in much the same way as a novelist or playwright presents his character. This may result in a fiction of over-simplification, yet it appears as an inevitable tendency. Then, to return to our caseworker, there is gradually formed a picture of her client, a picture that may vary somewhat, but which neverthe-less becomes perceptually characteristic, so that as interviews and meetings progress she comes to expect a certain pattern, to perceive the manifested behaviour as forming a particular organisation.

Experimental Study. An experiment which demonstrates the nature of this composite picture that we form of others was performed by the same author from whom we have just quoted.[41] Two groups of students were each given a list of qualities said to belong to one person. The list of the first group contained the qualities: intelligent, skillful, industrious, *warm*, determined, practical, cautious. The list for the second group contained the same traits as the first except for the substitution of *cold* for the adjective "warm". The two groups of students were then asked to write sketches of the person depicted with these adjectives, and to select from a list of traits the terms that they regarded as most appropriate to the impression that they had formed. What can be called the "warm" group of students thought the imaginary person was wise, humorous, popular, and imaginative, while the "cold" group held just the opposite impressions. As the experi-menter concluded, the change in just the one quality produced a basic transformation in the whole impression, although it was noticed from the results that the "warm" person is not viewed more favourably in *all* respects. Extrapolating from this single experiment, it can be suggested in a tentative way that one strong trait may well override other traits. Thus one may pay attention to Newton's theological writings and Einstein's comments on sociology on the strength of their prestige in the realm of physical science, although they would be entirely disregarded if they had been written by others, and although they are not remembered after a period of time. Similarly a first impression of confident bonhomie may well have the effect of ascribing qualities to a

[41] Asch, S. E. "Forming impressions of Personality". *J. Abn. Soc. Psychol.* 1946, *41*, 258.

person with that particular type of geniality which we ordinarily associate with that trait, and of omitting other qualities which we do *not* usually associate with it.

JUDGEMENT OF PERSONALITY

Having now discussed some of the ways in which impressions are formed, we now come to some of the phenomena involved in the actual judgement of others. It is not necessary to stress that this is basic for those who have to make decisions at first hand, or even to make an assessment over a period of time. One might almost say that impression formation and judgement go hand in hand. It is difficult for most people merely to record an impression and leave it at that; more likely than not there is involved some measure of critique in addition.

Judgemental Effects. There are some well known judgemental effects which can be listed. The best known of these is the so-called halo effect. This is an assessment based on a fairly general impression of either badness or goodness, and this rating creeps into other ratings. In other words the general impression over-flows into and overrides any specific impression. We saw an example of this in the instance of Newton and Einstein. To give another example—the habitual criminal is continually regarded with suspicion, a negative halo certainly, yet still a halo effect. In many ways this particular effect can be a stumbling-block when a careful and impartial valuation has to be made. It is therefore as well to follow Allport[42] in methods of diminishing this effect.

He catalogues seven different ways. "(a) by specific warning against it, (b) by employing distinctive and well-defined variables, (c) by using alert and trained judges, (d) by avoiding characterial and censorial variables, (e) by so varying the presentation of the qualities to be rated that a fresh and independent consideration of each is demanded, (f) by avoiding haste and perfunctoriness in making the ratings, and (g) by averaging together the ratings of several judges so that to some degree the prejudices of the several judges will cancel one another." Many of these warnings apply to situations where there is a team of judges; the individual, though, can profit from the general tenor of the methods.

[42] Allport, G. W. *Personality.*

A second effect, which has been called by Guildford[43] the logical error, is one in which certain traits are judged to go inevitably with other traits. Again this is an instance of the black and white, either-or type of categorisation to which many people are prone. For instance if a person is judged stupid he may also be labelled lazy, or if a man is judged vindictive he may also be thought to be "touchy". Such a logical error has the more force as more likely than not it may have been found to be correct in the past. A third effect in the judgement of impressions of others is the leniency effect. Here the tendency is to regard others high in favourable traits and low in unfavourable traits. The nursery rhyme reflects this when it says, "There was a little girl . . . when she was good, she was very, very, good, And when she was bad, she was horrid."

Causal Factors. Such are the general types of effects which inevitably colour the overall impression and affect judgement accordingly. We now have to consider some of the causal factors, and to see which of these make for accuracy of judgement. One of the most noticeable points is that a trait is the more easily judged if it is manifested in a sequence. Bender and Hastorf[44] found that people could predict better the responses of their friends to items of social situations than to items regarding social feelings. This was because not only are "social situations" more visible than "socal feelings", but also because it was in a context. This is largely common sense and is what one would expect. If a person loses his temper and throws things about, it is patently easier to judge that he is angry than when a person is containing himself and one is uncertain as to his real feelings. What makes inference more difficult are the cases where a gesture is either not known or misinterpreted. A pursing of the lips may be taken either as a sign of impatience or it may represent thoughtfulness. If a gesture signifies surprise in one culture and rudeness in another, the cross-correspondence of emotional manifestations must first be learned.

[43] Guildford, J. P. *Psychometric Methods.* McGraw-Hill, 1936. This error was originally drawn attention to by Newcomb.
[44] Bender, I. E. and Hastorf, A. H. "The Perception of Persons: Forecasting another person's responses on three personality scales". *J. Abn. Soc. Psychol.* 1950, *45*, 556.

Of prime importance is the effect of the relationship between the judge and judged. The interaction doubtless influences the type of trait to be estimated. In social work this is eminently so: an almoner is looking at her charge with a view to whether he will be able to withstand the vicissitudes of post-hospital life; the psychiatric social worker is geared for evidence of abnormality; the family caseworker has an eye for social and family relationships. Many of these traits overlap and many are sought for by one judge; the point is that judgement is made from the particular standpoint of the assessor, he is looking for clues that will elucidate this standpoint. Bruner and Tagiuri[45] have emphasised this point in their consideration of a mechanic in the Army, who comes into interaction with two men. The first is a fellow mechanic, who forms his impressions in terms of whether the other man is a good mechanic, cheerful and a "nice guy". The second man is an officer who is looking for evidence of reliability, initiative and courage. In other words, both men are seeking for impressions that involve the relationship with the mechanic.

There is a great deal of literature on the subject of interaction between judged and judge; the more important items will be selected. First, there is the actual relationship. Similarity in terms of age, sex, background and complexity tends to increase accuracy of judgement. Second, role relationships is another important item. It is known that lecturers' judgements of their students were biased by knowledge of their academic ability (similar to the "halo effect"). Degree of acquaintance and affection makes for more favourable ratings. All this is still really connected with the positive side of the halo effect, and again is what is to be expected. The mother who defends her errant offspring after his third charge, by stating that after all he really is a good boy, fits into this side of the judgemental picture.

First Impressions. Such relationships are by definition over a a period of time. It may be asked, to complete the rest of the picture, what is the effect of a first impression? A first impression very often has the poignancy that successive responses lack. Very

---

[45] Bruner, J. S. and Tagiuri, R. "The Perception of People". In Lindzey, G. *Handbook of Social Psychology*, Vol. II. This chapter includes most of the references alluded to in this section.

often this is born of necessity. A candidate coming up for inter-view has only the one opportunity to make good; his selectors have *their* only chance. Also a good impression may make a somewhat lasting effect. The experimental evidence of this is slight however. Dailey[46] reports that the formation of a first impression may have the result of rigidifying and impairing later judgements.

Qualities of a Good Judge. All such speculation can be over-shadowed by the particular qualities of the referee himself. What are the endowments that make for a good judge? Doubtless there are many, according to time and situation; only three will be mentioned, namely detachment, æsthetic sensitivity, and ex-perience. Disinterestedness, in the sense of impartiality and lack of emotional involvedness, is always preferable. It has been found experimentally that judges who became emotional in the process of making a judgement did least well. Also Taft[47] compiled a list of adjectives from numerous people which was adjudged to characterise a good assessor: the list, containing words such as calm, quiet, realistic, logical, serious, and sincere, arrow the direction in which an impartial observer is found. With regard to the second quality, æsthetic sensitivity, there is some disagree-ment. F. H. Allport[48] was of the opinion that it was of prime importance, but Taft, on the basis of research, found this did not hold with sophisticated artistic interests, only with simple æsthetic sensitivity. As regards the third quality, experience, there is little available evidence. *Prima facie* one would suppose it to be basic, but it is the *type* of experience that matters. Perhaps the most important item in this concerns the experience of a particu-lar culture. To cite Bruner and Tagiuri yet once more, they sug-gest that a knowledge of culture pressures increases the predictive power of a judge. Certainly a knowledge of the gestures, habits and interests of a person of another culture increases the possi-bilities of not drawing faulty inferences because of the fallacy of

---

[46] Dailey, C. A. "Some factors influencing the accuracy of understanding per-sonality". Unpublished doctoral dissertation, 1951. Quoted by Bruner and Tagiuri. *op. cit.*

[47] Taft, R. See Bruner and Tagiuri, but also "Some characteristics of good Judges of others". *Brit. J. Psychol.* 1956, 19.

[48] Allport, F. H. *Social Psychology.* Houghton Mifflin. 1924. Again cited by Bruner and Tagiuri.

making conclusions within the framework of one's own culture. A difficulty, one might add, which is by no means that simple to overcome without considerable experience of another culture.

PERCEPTION OF THE ILL

We began this section with a quotation from John Clare, showing that illness can colour one's perceptions of other people and of life generally. This, though, has repercussions far beyond the perceptions of the patient himself. There is his family to be considered—how do they regard illness and what are their reactions?

Venereal Disease. Before we consider the family aspect, there is the patient himself to be discussed. One really has to regard unusual cases in order to get a picture of what this can mean. Thus, as an example, Snelling[49] observed the reactions of women in a V.D. clinic. As might have been expected these patients were hypersensitive. Snelling noted that a patient, in her desire for anonymity, will often put the most foolish constructions on any aside remarks or glances given to her. In addition, "her normal standards of judgement will be shaken. She may expect unprofessional conduct of us all (i.e. the workers in the clinic), for instance gossip, when in other circumstances she would know better." In such an illness to which is attached a social opprobrium, it is a very delicate matter to present a helpful attitude. Snelling makes some proposals for this: showing no surprise at the patient's attendances, implying that other people have been in the same position, lack of interest in personal matters of the patient, and allowing contradictory or variable statements to pass unquestioned.

Blindness and Deafness. If we turn to the perceptions of blind and deaf people, there is not of course any social censure, but there is the concomitant aspect of social relations. Anderson[50] cites two anecdotal examples of the misconceptions that ordinary people can have about the blind: in the first case a railway conductor

[49] Snelling, J. "A Study of some emotional problems in a V.D. Clinic". *Social Work* 1946, *3*, 275.
[50] Anderson, D. K. "The Social Caseworker's relation to concepts of blindness". *Social Casework* 1950, *31*, 416.

called for a wheel-chair for a young blind woman who was travelling alone, and in the second case a waitress asked the friend of a blind man, in the presence of the latter, if he, the blind person, would like some cream in his coffee. These may be odd examples, yet there is no denying the strange fact that normally healthy people are embarassed when they meet a case of physical handicap. In addition there is the well known fact that deaf people are often rated to be stupid.

Guilt and Shame. Where there is a social atmosphere of guilt or shame about the illness, as in the case with venereal disease, the situation is further complicated. We might take as a further example of this the instance of the reactions of relatives to mental disease in their spouses or children. Rogers[51] made a study of the reactions of married couples to the fact that one of the pair was a patient in a psychiatric clinic. There were a number of reactions: there was the spouse who was doubtful and fearful, and who assumed a disinterestedness, and was sometimes even hostile; others who were more superficial in reaction; and there were still others who had some awareness of the need for assistance in the problem of their husband or wife. Somewhat similar is the report made by Freeman[52] in his work with families of patients in mental hospitals, or who had returned from mental hospitals. He finds three distinct groups among these families. The first, which need not be discussed, comprises those who take an intelligent concern about the patient and his problem. The second group include those in whom there is a problem attitude, yet not so strong as to be incapable of being changed. The third group comprises the cases where the problem attitude is rigid and unchangeable. With regard to the second and third groups, Freeman notes that they usually have emotional disturbances of their own and are apt to lean heavily on the patient when he returns to the home, or even when he is still hospitalised. Whereas the second group can modify their attitudes and problems, the third group is characterised by a return to the old way of conduct. Freeman describes such people with related advice for the psychiatric

[51] Rogers, P. A. "Casework with spouses of psychiatric patients". *Smith College Studies in Social Work*, 1946, *16*, 265.
[52] Freeman, H. "Casework with families of mental hospital patients". *Social Casework*. 1947, *28*, 107.

social worker, "In such instances, when the patient is allowed to go home, it must be expected that the relative is going to insist upon returning to or keeping up the old emotional patterns that existed prior to hospitalisation. This should be carefully evaluated in terms of how much the patient's condition can absorb. This is particularly important because these relatives often place the most intensive pressure upon the doctors to have the patient released."

Individual reactions, such as in the case of the families mentioned above, really indicate appearances of a much wider context, that is of the influence of social perception. Our individual perceptions, of the nature that is at present being considered, are strongly tinged with the hall-mark of the particular group to which we belong. It so happens that in our culture, or at least in particular sub-sections of our culture, mental illness has a definite stigmata. The individual's perception is encapsulated in the group's perception, the group that is to say to which he bears allegiance. The implicit values which the group holds strongly effects the way in which a member of it will "perceive" a situation or an event. This we have already noted in the section on "Social Perception". It is stressed again here to include matters concerning definite types of illness.

Evaluation. It would be insufficient to terminate this section by reference to outstanding illnesses or cases alone. This has been done with the intention of bringing out the factor of perception. It is clear that all illness brings with it definite variances of perceiving, by the patient himself, as well as by his relatives and friends. Thus it is clear that surgery presents difficulties of its own kind. But to delve into this and similar conditions is to move away from particular points into generalities. It is of no consequence to know that a patient with jaundice looks upon the world with his proverbial eye. To be of note we must look for further facts of a more fruitful nature. What might be termed "social diseases" provide in fact just this, but it must be added that this is a field in which further research, including a wide variety of illnesses and under a wide range of conditions and social atmospheres, is very much required.

V

COMMUNICATION

THERE need not be very deep reflection to realise that communication, in one form or another, enters into all our human activities. There is a form of communication at an unconscious level of bodily activity where internal processes are constantly adapting to one another. When a person moves his arm there is a finely elaborated system of communication between his brain and his arm that enables him to perform this simple action. When somebody is pricked by a pin there is started a channel of impulses beginning at the level of his skin and continuing to the brain. We have also to remind ourselves that the name given to those chemical substances which are secreted by the endocrine glands and are carried by the blood to initiate activity to another organ—hormones—are the Greek name for messengers. Apart from the internal environment of our bodies and the information selected from the outside world, there is the daily interchange of information between people. This can be verbal or non-verbal, the former relying on language and the latter mainly on gestures. Lastly society may be said to be organised through communication, by means of correspondence, telephone exchanges, radio, television and the like.

There are basically three elements in the social process of communication: there is the person who passes on the information, the information itself, and the person who receives it; in short, the communicator, the communiqué, and the communicant. In this Chapter we shall discuss some of the aspects of the interactions of these elements, paying special attention to the distortion of information.

Perception and Communication. The subject of communication cannot be separated from the subject of perception. The two are integrated: that is only communicated which has been perceived, and that which is perceived depends very much upon the input of information. A classical experiment demonstrating this latter point was carried out with a set of ambiguous figures[1] given to a group of subjects to reproduce immediately after presentation. Half of these subjects were told that a particular figure was one object, the other half that it represented another object. Thus one drawing was said to be a crescent moon to the first half, and the second half were told that it was the letter C. The actual figure was intermediate between these two possibilities, and was drawn ambiguous on purpose. The reproductions made showed clearly that the verbal label had a strong influence. Those subjects that had been informed that the drawing was that of a crescent moon made their reproductions more like this than the original. The subjects that had been told that it was the letter C, depicted their drawings by a strong resemblance to the third letter of the alphabet. This experiment shows how language affects what we see. The full force of this feature will become more apparent in the following sections.

Modes of Communication. One can talk about communication in the manner in which information is transmitted. A one-way communication channel is represented by the types of mass media, newspapers, radio, films and television. Here something is transmitted to thousands of people; readers, listeners and viewers. Although in these cases there is an indirect response by virtue of the fact that people write letters to the newspapers, ring up the B.B.C., and that the outgoing information is sometimes modified because of this, there is no clear two-way process as in a telephone conversation. A two-way channel can be characterised by the latter example, or by a conversation between two people, or by an exchange of letters. In these instances there is a constant stream of information going back and forth, each separate message being constructed in response to the previous message. Thirdly there can be a network of communication in which a number of people are involved, as in a discussion group, or in a chain of neighbours relaying gossip over garden fences.

---

[1] Carmichael, L., Hogan, H. P. and Walter, A. A. "An experimental study of the effect of language on the reproduction of visually perceived form." *J. exp. Psychol.* 1932, *15*, 73.

The form of the network can be of importance in some cases. An experiment with a group of five people illustrates the possibilities.[2] The five were arranged in different forms of communication networks, by being placed in separate cubicles set in various ways. The five subjects were able to get in touch with one another by written messages, but the arrangement of their ability to communicate with one another varied. In one form the cubicles were arranged in a circle, so that each member could correspond with his neighbours, that is to say only two people. In a second pattern the cubicles were arranged in a straight line. In this linear form the middle member had the advantage over the others, as he was the only person who could not only communicate directly with the persons either side of him, but the extreme members of the group were only one remove away. The second and fourth members could relay messages to people either side of them but one member was two stages away. The third type of pattern, common to the Army or to a business organisation, was the inverted Y form. There were three sub-arrangements of this type. The formation could either be fixed so that messages could be sent in a straight line for the first three members and then split to the fourth and fifth, or the split could come at the stage of the second member, or the first person could send directions. to all the others. Now these five subjects, placed in their various arrangements of cubicles, were given simple problems to solve jointly. Their efficiency could be measured by the number of messages passed, as well as by the errors made and the time taken. It was found that a problem was solved most efficiently when the cubicles were arranged either in a straight line or in the inverted Y pattern. These were the forms in which the arrangement was least "democratic". There was a definite leader in these forms, who could direct the messages without too much contagion from others. However this was not the only effect, and a trend was observed which detracted from the gain of efficiency. In the linear and inverted Y forms the group as a whole was dissatisfied. The circular pattern was marked by a feeling of enjoyment in the problem, although this way resulted in the most amount of errors and the longest time. The feeling of satisfaction with this order of the cubicles was due to the fact that everybody was partici-

---

[2] Leavitt, H. J. "Some effects of certain communication patterns on group performance". *J. Abnorm. Soc. Psychol.* 1951, *46*, 38.

pating in the project; the members were happy because they felt that they were all equally contributing to the problem. Where the onus of direction fell just upon one member, and the rest were compelled to follow blindly, there was the atmosphere of "feeling out of things". Hence although there was a reduction of errors there was also a feeling of discontent. If we can extrapolate this laboratory experiment to situations in businesses and factories, the moral is plain. The satisfied worker is in fact a collaborator. Loss of communication may pay dividends in increased efficiency in the short run, but may lead to dissatisfaction in the long run.

SOCIAL EFFECTS

We have already noted in the previous Chapter how society and culture can influence the selection of what is perceived. We have now to discuss the social effects upon the *transmission* of what is perceived.

REMEMBERING

The two chief ways of remembering are by recall and recognition. One may recall a name of a friend either by vocalising it or writing it down on paper, reproducing the name, or one might forget the name yet be able to recognise it within a list of other names. In this section we shall concentrate on the social factors in recall.[3]

Experimental Method. There are two ways of studying this aspect of recall. The first is called the Method of Repeated Reproduction. A person is given a story or a simple drawing or a prose passage involving an argument which he is asked to study. After a quarter of an hour he is asked to reproduce whatever he has seen, and then further reproductions are made at increasing intervals. The time period of the reproductions can last over months and even years. The second method, called the Method of Serial Reproduction, is similar to the first except that instead of the same subject reproducing the material over and over again, his reproduction is given to another subject who passes it on to a third

[3] From Bartlett, F. C. *Remembering. A Study in Experimental and Social Psychology.* Cambridge University Press 1932. The studies included further experimental methods and other types of material than the ones referred to here.

subject and so on. With verbal passages each subject was allowed to read the story twice, while there was an interval of a quarter to half an hour, in which the subject was kept mentally engaged, before the material was reproduced to the next person.

Common to both of the methods used by Bartlett was a translation of a North American folk-tale called "The War of the Ghosts". The choice of this type of narrative was made because it originated from a different culture and social environment than that to which the subjects belonged; the story itself lacked obvious rational order, and thirdly the dramatic nature of the tale was likely to arouse vivid visual imagery in some subjects. Also as the author phrased it: "I had also in mind the general problem of what actually happens when a popular story travels about from one social group to another, and thought that possibly the use of this story might throw some light upon the general conditions of transformation under such circumstances."

With the first method it was found that although there was little accuracy of literal reproduction, the general outline of the story was remembered fairly persistently. What was of some importance were the processes of rationalisation. The material was reduced to a form that was able to be assimilated in a satisfying manner to the subject. Logical inconsequencies or incoherencies in the story were reconstructed; the tale was given a general setting appropriate to an educated reader or listener. What Bartlett has called an "effort after meaning" loomed largely in these reproductions. To quote from the study, "It could be said that there is a constant effort to get the maximum possible of meaning into the material presented." With the reconstruction of details the process of rationalisation is due to the particular characteristics of the subject. Furthermore names, phrases and events in the narrative tend to be altered to fit in with current forms of the particular social group to which the subject belongs.

In Serial Reproduction there can be very great alterations to the material. "Epithets are changed into their opposites; incidents and events are transposed; names and numbers rarely survive intact for more than a few reproductions; opinions and conclusions are reversed—nearly every possible variation seems as if it can take place, even in a relatively short series." A notable item is "conventionalisation". The individual characteristics of the story become lost and the arguments and opinions in the narrative are reconstructed into conventional views. The conventional views, that is to say, of the transmitter. Rationalisation again takes place, and there is also a tendency for abstract points to be lost in favour of the concrete.

These experiments bring out very forcibly the fact that remembering is influenced by the tendencies within a culture or society or group. When these tendencies are strong the material is likely to be constructive and inventive.

RUMOUR

The second part of Shakespeare's *King Henry the Fourth* opens with a speech by a character painted full of tongues called Rumour, in which he describes himself "as a pipe blown by surmises, jealousies, conjectures". The picture is fairly apt. Rumours are made up from elements of hostility, fear and wishes. They reflect the tension of the community; in particular they appear to be a barometer of group hostility. Allport and Postman[4] have defined the functions of rumour as "explaining and relieving emotional tensions felt by individuals". Rumours at once are a result of emotional tensions and contribute towards them. In times of crisis the critical faculty is diminished and people are inclined to believe those tales which fit into their hopes or fears, likes or dislikes. These stories, becoming even more distorted in further circulation help to sustain and provoke further a feeling of tension. The process tends to be circular; the acceptance of a rumour relieves the tension, but the very relief predisposes a person to acknowledge the rumour.

The Experimental Study of Rumour. The method used in rumour studies is similar to Serial Reproduction. A slide is shown on a screen, illustrating a semi-dramatic picture with a great many details. An audience can see this screen. But the chosen subjects who are brought on the stage cannot see the picture, and are only told about it. In the case of the first subject either one of the audience or an experimenter describes the picture to him. Thereafter the first subject tells the second subject, who tells the third, and so on. All the time the audience see the picture on the screen and can thus observe the gradual stages of deterioration.

[4] Allport, G. W. and Postman, L. J. "The Basic Psychology of Rumor". In Newcomb and Hartley: *Readings in Social Psychology*. See also Allport and Postman's book *The Psychology of Rumor*. Holt 1947.

The effect of having an audience at all can be assessed by using a group of subjects without one. The general influence of an audience was to make the subjects more cautious.

As a rumour circulates, it becomes shorter and more concise, the more easier to grasp. There are less and less words used and details remembered. This feature is called "levelling". For example with one picture described to five successive subjects, the first reproduction retained 68% of the details, the second 54%, and the final one only 30%. A reciprocal feature is called "sharpening". With this process a number of items are picked out from a larger portion. One particular item may catch the mind of the listener and he builds up a whole story around this solitary point. There are at least six features which make for sharpening. An odd word may be seized on and retained throughout the series, although it has but little importance in the story. It is similar with familiar symbols, such as a church and a cross, although in the picture depicted they are of little note. Temporal sharpening takes place in the form that the present moment is of the most importance. If a story is told in the past tense it can quickly become converted to the present. Non-moving things tend to start moving. The authors report as a common occurrence that stationary trains are reproduced as moving. Size is yet another aspect of sharpening. An object that is very large is retained throughout the reproductions merely because of its size. Lastly labels tend to persist—"One picture is usually introduced by some version of the statement, 'This is a battle scene', and this label persists throughout the series of reproductions."

A third feature is "assimilation". This is the effect produced on the content by all the existing habits of thought. The listener's habits and outlook absorbs the new content and gives it a particular shape. This is similar to what Bartlett has called "conventionalisation". There are a number of factors by which assimilation can take place. There can be an assimilation to a principal theme. There is a reconstruction of details around a central point. If a battle incident is shown then more buildings are reported to be demolished than there are actually in the picture. Expectation is another important assimilating mechanism. It corresponds very much to the stereotype which we have already discussed in the previous chapter. An example of this occurs very often in a picture of a white man holding a razor talking to a negro. Before very long in the series of reproductions, when shown to white subjects, it is the negro that is holding the instrument. Things are represented by how it is thought they "ought" to be rather than as they are. With the case of the negro picture, there is the added assimilation to prejudice. It was found that negro subjects nearly always avoided mentioning colour.

These three factors of levelling, sharpening and assimilation interact and function simultaneously. Their net result is called "the embedding process" Allport and Postman have summarised the results of these experiments thus: "What seems to occur in all our experiments and in all related studies is that each subject finds the outer stimulus-world far too hard to grasp and retain in its objective character. For his personal uses, it must be recast to fit not only his span of comprehension and his span of retention, but likewise, his own personal needs and interests. What was outer becomes inner; what was objective becomes subjective. In telling a rumor, the kernel of objective information that he received has become so embedded into his own dynamic mental life that the product is chiefly one of projection. Into the rumor, he projects the deficiencies of his retentive processes, as well as his own effort to engender meaning upon an ambiguous field, and the product reveals much of his own emotional needs, including his anxieties, hates and wishes. When several rumor-agents have been involved in this embedding process, the net result of the serial reproduction reflects the lowest common denominator of cultural interest, of memory span, and of group sentiment and prejudice."

TESTIMONY

There is nothing so shattering to the belief in the infallibility of human observation and memory than a study of the evidence regarding testimony. Time and time again it has been demonstrated how easily people fail to observe; how they are misled during observation, and how difficult it is to keep an incident in mind untrammelled for longer than a few hours. And all this is prior to the actual reporting of an incident, a further factor which introduces with it the problems of the choice of words and the errors due to being questioned in a certain way. There is then a three-fold sequence involved in testimony: the initial observation, retention, and communication. We shall provide examples of each of these stages.

MAL-OBSERVATION

Let us begin by considering a typical study, an experiment arranged in a lecture room.[5] Two students were seen to behave in a disorderly fashion during the lecture, whereupon the lecturer asked the rest of the class to write down a detailed account of the incident which had lasted only a few minutes. A full account would have contained ten essential points, yet the average number reported was only three and a half. In a further study, a three-minute film was shown to a collection of schoolgirls, and then to adults, after which they were asked a number of questions. One question was whether the lamp had been on the table or hanging from the ceiling. Each subject reported one of these alternatives, although in fact there had been neither lamp nor table. What is disturbing in this example, with relevance to testimony, is not so much the omission of noting that something is absent, as the readiness to deny this in favour of a positive substitute. Most of us would be hard pressed if we were suddenly asked for the pattern of the wall-paper in our bed-room (the very familiarity of it seems to block the recall), but it is interesting to speculate whether we would provide an answer to this question when in fact there was no wall-paper. This has connections with the way in which the question is formulated, a feature which will be taken up later.

An Experimental "Crime". It is difficult to simulate the conditions of real life, where testimony takes place with all the attendant qualities of surprise and emotion. Nevertheless experiments have been attempted, a typical study being one where a "crime" was presented before one hundred and fifty girls.[6] A class of girls had been listening to their instructor talking for a quarter of an hour when suddenly a boy appeared followed by two pursuers. All three rushed on to the stage in full view of the audience, overturning furniture, making a great amount of noise, shouting

[5] Wolters, A. W. P. *The Evidence of Our Senses.* Methuen 1933.
[6] Vickery, K., and Brooks, L. M. "Time-spaced reporting of a 'crime' witnessed by college girls". *J. Crim. Law Criminol.* 1938, *29*, 371.

and exclaiming. The period of the "crime" lasted for only one and a half minutes. There were three stages in the interrogation. Immediately after the incident the instructor rebuked the boys and asked the class to write out a description of what they had observed. A week later there was an unannounced questionnaire form given to the girls demanding answers to questions about the incident, couched in different styles. Finally, seven weeks later, again with no warning, there was a second test in the same form as the previous questionnaire. The results showed first of all that there was very little agreement between the correct statements made in the free description of the incident and the two direct question forms given one week and seven weeks later. It seemed, too, to make no difference if one "witness" could recall many items as against another who could recall only a few: the ratio of correct to false statements in either was about the same. It is interesting also to note that there was no relationship between the mental ability of the observers or the degree of neuroticism and the amount of evidence volunteered. As regards the actual observation, it was found that the ability to describe the "criminals" was inferior to the reporting of the action itself, and although the scene of the incident was very familiar to the audience, the ability to describe it was the poorest of the lot. This incident had been well prepared beforehand, and the boys had been rehearsed in their actions and exclamations. Also the dimensions of the scene were known, and the time of the incident calculated. Although the period of the occurrence was very short there was a very poor response in attempts to estimate the duration of it. Estimations of distance were also very varied and inaccurate. Of the description of the boys, there was a tendency to be able to judge age better than physical characteristics. In particular the observers tended to underestimate height.

An Experimental Identification Parade. The above account was an attempt to approximate to real life conditions. Another attempt,[7] though this time aimed at identification akin to police methods of identification parades, was made with four groups of students under different conditions. The test was that of the identification of a stranger, dressed as a workman, who walked across the

[7] Brown, H. B. "An Experience in Identification testimony". *J. Crim. Law Criminol.* 1934, *25*, 621.

classroom. He passed the instructor's desk, played around with the radiator, made an audible question about the heat, retraced his steps and departed. Sixteen days later this man was put up together with five other men of the same general appearance and clothing. These men were lined up in random order before the students who were asked to indicate on a questionnaire the man they had seen on the previous occasion, together with the degree of confidence (on a five point scale) that they felt in this judgement. The first group of thirty students, who were accustomed to these surprise experiments, was the most accurate. Seventy-six per cent of the group made a correct identification. The second group, of sixty-four students, had had no previous experience, and of these just over seventeen per cent were unable to make a correct identification. With the third group, composed of sixteen students, there was a change in the experimental conditions. Only five men appeared before them, the one they had seen enter their classroom being the missing man. Nevertheless over sixty-two per cent of the class identified a wrong man, only four stating that the correct man was absent. With the fourth group of seventeen students, there was again a change. These students had not been in the class and thus had not witnessed the incident. Yet they were asked to identify a man they had never actually seen, and in fact nearly thirty per cent "remembered" an incident which they had never witnessed.

Experiments like these could be multiplied. The examples given illustrate only too well how difficult it is to achieve any unanimity among a number of observers, and how flimsy a picture the final verdict is for any outside person whose business it is to gain the truth of what "actually" happened. It must be emphasised that this is no question as to the honesty or the credibility of witnesses. Where these factors come into play then the story assumes further elaborations. These are matters of psychological interest peculiar to the ordinary person. Training of observation no doubt corrects many of these errors and omissions, but only a very few people are so trained, and they do not make up the huge bulk of people who stand in the witness box day after day and give their observations.

RETENTION

We have already seen, in the previous section, the properties of remembering and especially the social influence of the content retained. In taking up the subject again from the point of view of considering what is retained of an initial observation between the time that it is made and when it is reported, or in addition, when the same observation is reported for a second or third time, we see once more the paucity of human memory. In the experiment described above of the "crime" enacted before the college girls, a further question was asked, one week afterwards, as to the date of the incident. At this stage eighty-six per cent of the class remembered the date with accuracy, yet when the same question was again asked in the seven week later test, eighty per cent could not answer this question, and of those who responded with some date, none gave the correct one.

That memory can play odd tricks is well know. Wolters[8] gives an account of how he went one day to photograph a doorway in an old house that he had often seen before. When he arrived at the place there was no doorway to be seen, and he realised that the "doorway" had been an addition of his own. As he himself put it: "The 'memory' was as clear and as confidently held as could be desired, and but for the test he would have remained convinced that he had seen it in a particular spot. This is a gross case of supplementation, sufficient to inform us that much that we 'remember' is an involuntary creation. Notice, too, that confidence that our memory is correct affords no indication whatever of its reliability."

The previous accounts of the errors in remembering described in the last section of the work of Bartlett and of the psychology of rumour, renders further elaboration here unnecessary. It is only raised now to emphasise that testimony is not often immediate after the observation. There elapses a period between observation and recall in which all the known psychological factors can interfere with the initial recording of the event. As very few people write down what they have witnessed immediately after the event, it is to be assumed that the distortion is liable to be magnified in proportion to the time when they report it. A long period provides occasion for all the effects of rationalisation and conventionalisation which Bartlett discovered. A person then begins to report not so much what he remembers of the incident as what he "remembers what he remembers".

[8] *Op. cit.*

REPORTING

We are now concerned with the manner in which an incident is recorded and with the type of questions used to discover what has happened. In brief there are two main methods of enquiry: the witness can be asked to write down or narrate a free description of what he had observed; or else this is found out by asking him questions, either orally or in written form in the manner of a questionnaire. Stern,[9] one of the leading early investigators on the reliability of testimony, made three tests with these two methods of extracting information. In the first case there was a picture briefly exposed, in the second test an event was staged, and in the third test written material was used. The observer had to write down what he had seen: in the first method he merely had to write in the form of a narrative what he had witnessed, with the second method he was required to answer specific questions in the form of a deposition. The deposition form proved to have the drawback that it depended upon the way the question was asked. A plain determinative type of question—Did the woman cross the road? for instance, was much less confusing than the implicative type, What road did the woman cross?, in which it is already assumed that she did in fact cross the road. We shall have more to say about this later. Of the narrative form, statements which were sworn were more accurate than unsworn statements, indicating that the procedure of taking the oath in court has the merit of making a person more careful in what he says.

It might be asked what happens in those cases where both types of enquiry are held, the free narrative and the deposition in sequence? This has been answered at least in one case by the fact that the deposition is influenced by the writing of a narrative prior to it, in that the number of correct responses is increased and the number of "don't know" responses is decreased. Yet there is no appreciable alteration in incorrect answers. This study also showed with the reverse case, where the narrative follows the deposition, that the alteration is more serious.

Stern found that the testimony of a witness shows a decrease in reliability of about thirty per cent from giving a coherent report to answers in cross-examination. He pointed out that the witness has

---

[9] See Stern, W. "Abstract of Lectures on the psychology of testimony and the study of Individuality". *Amer. J. Psychol.* 1910, *21*, 270; and "The Psychology of Testimony". *J. Abn. Soc. Psychol.* 1939, *34*, 3.

a tendency in cross-examination to prefer to give an incorrect answer rather than confess that he does not know. It is very difficult to generalise here from different experimental evidence. It may be that the kind of event witnessed, its significance for the observer, the atmosphere in which information is extracted, and last but not least the nature of the observer, all hold equal influence on the method of interrogation. Until more is known about the bearing of these variables, it is impossible to give ready conclusions.

Form of the Question. What can be shown with some force is the effect of the way in which a question is couched. The influence of the "leading question" is notorious, and it is not very difficult to show that for questions such as "Was the man not old?" the answer is more likely to be Yes than No if the witness is not sure. Similarly as Moore[10] states, when one asks: "Didn't the wrecked car skid before it stopped?" the question is liable to decrease the caution of the witness.

A systematic attempt to discover the effects of the suggestiveness of questions was made by Muscio[11] some years ago. He displayed to numerous groups a silent film, then asked questions which were cast in eight different forms, as below.

	1.	Did you see a....?
Subjective	2.	Did you see the....?
	3.	*Didn't* you see a....?
	4.	*Didn't* you see the....?
	5.	Was there a....?
Objective	6.	*Wasn't* there a....?
	7.	Was the K, *m* or *n*? (e.g. was the man, *bearded* or *clean shaven*?)
	8.	Was the K, *m*? (e.g. was the man, *bearded*?)

Muscio found that the negative form of a question—*Didn't* you see, or *wasn't* there . . . , was always more productive of suggestibility than the positive form. Similarly the definite article—

[10] Moore, E. H. "Elements of error in testimony". *J. App. Psych.* 1935, *19*, 447.
[11] Muscio, B. "The Influence of the form of a question". *Brit. J. Psychol.* 1916, *8*, 351.

Was *the* car there, aroused more suggestibility than the question was *a* car there, using the indefinite article. Muscio also noted that questions involving personal references were always more productive than others.

So much for the errors arising from the form of the question. Quite apart from this is the fact that verbal formulation has its own intrinsic pitfalls. Stern[12] describes two ways in which errors can develop in this respect. When testimony is given over a period of time at successive intervals, the expressions of the previous accounts are better remembered than the initial accident. As we have noted before, there is the "memory of a memory". Stern makes the comment that the "verbal form gradually becomes *stereotyped*—a sign that in place of pictorial remembrance of objects, verbal remembrance has been introduced". The second way in which error is introduced, according to Stern, lies in the ambiguity of language. It might so happen in a second or third account of what had been witnessed that a reproduced word will elicit a different mental image. Stern gives the example of a subject describing the picture of an artist moving with the poetic phrase "a painter is approaching the gateway of a new life". A few weeks later all that was retained was the word "gateway" but its metaphorical context was lost. As a consequence of this he wrote: "A moving van is passing through a narrow gateway", thus embroidering around the remembered word a different and more rationalising context. In the actual picture there had been no gateway at all.

Thus we see that there are three sources of mistakes at this stage of testimony. There is the factor of the form of interrogation; there is the difficulty arising from cross-examination of the way a question is framed; and there is the inherent drawbacks due to the use of language itself. If we couple on to these the deficiencies of observation already noted, it is a small wonder that anything is ever accurately reported at all. Perhaps it is not.

RECOMMENDATIONS

We have given this section the context of legal testimony, partly because the experimental work has this background, and partly because of the audience for which this is intended. It must be borne in mind, however, that the nature of testimony covers

[12] *Op. cit.*

an area of interest wider than the police courts. Whenever somebody reports some place or object about which nobody else has
seen or known, and about which he cannot give any other evidence
than that he has been there or seen it, then the psychology of
testimony comes into play. One has in mind certain examples.
When Stanley returned from having discovered Livingstone, he
was not at first believed. The evidence current in psychic research
pertaining to apparitions and the like has to be looked at from the
point of honesty and suggestion. People who say they have
spoken with occupants of Flying Saucers are clearly not believed.
Even quite respectable observations in Science are taken with
sceptical regard if they seem fantastic or out of accordance with
the accustomed way of thinking; and until they can be repeated
by somebody else, or made plausible by logical reasoning, then
the psychology of testimony enters. The account of historians,
often giving completely different stories of the same battle, have
to be weighed from points of view of accessibility to the facts,
amount of prejudice, and so forth. In all these fields the prestige of
the witness occupies a large part. Thus if the Astronomer Royal
solemnly declares that he has seen the Loch Ness Monster, he
is more likely to be believed than somebody who is not known at
all. And although this is a classical fallacy, the *argumentum ad
verecundiam*, there is little doubt that it operates psychologically.

Given this larger context, the issue of testimony enters the subject of logic, and there are known arguments and suitable demonstrations to be learned from the logic of testimony. However we
shall not wander from the psychology of the subject, but keep to
the recommendations relevant to psychological mechanisms.

Stern, to quote him once more, drew up a list of the practical
consequences for law from an estimate of psychological investigations. The first consequence is a negative one, namely that the
reliance on witnesses' reports should be lessened. Another consequence, but this time a recommendation in a positive sense, is that
an inquisitor should assist in lowering the amount of falsification
by leaving more to spontaneous narration (it had been Stern's
finding that this was preferable to cross-examination) and making
his questions less suggestive. A third point has reference to the
problem of identification. He recommends that a person should
identify from a group of similar people, and not be asked in
effect "Was *this* the man you saw?" This is established procedure

now (Stern's article was published in 1910), but of course the key word is *similar*. It is not so simple to suddenly arrange for a number of like people to appear before a witness, and it is to be surmised how approximate identification parades are in this respect. Finally to summarise Stern's conclusions from his and others' investigations, we shall quote his estimation of the value of psychological experimentation. "Psychological experiments show what degree of confidence ought in general to be placed in particular classes of testimony. It teaches, for example, that colors to which particular attention has not been given are especially ill-remembered; that times of a few minutes are almost always considerably over-estimated; that the main outlines of an event, if they have been followed with attention and if the witness has not shared especially in the emotions involved, are commonly correctly reproduced; that on the contrary, things observed without attention are very liable to distortion (for this reason delayed reports with reference to the appearance or clothing of a person not carefully observed are for the most part worthless)."

Such is the evaluation of one of the pioneers of this branch of psychology. At a later date Wolters[13] considers it impossible to give specific advice, but recommends cautiously a few points. The advice is cautious because as he points out it is all very well to recommend to people what they should or should not observe and recall, but all such advice has the contingency of detachment which is least likely in scenes of accidents, and in fact in most cases where evidence would be needed. Given this uncertainty, he recommends that observers should put their attention on details and try to recall a few points. He advises against a great effort to remember when pressed for information, because this, as we have already noted before, encourages false elaboration. "Offer what comes naturally and clearly, and stifle any false pride that stands in the way of confessing ignorance."

As Wolters states, it is very difficult to give any advice. The detached "cool observer" or the "born witness" cannot be manufactured. If there is one over-all advice to be given, it is that when confronted with a situation where evidence might be needed, the observer should *immediately* write down everything that he has seen, trying to omit no detail. This does not help in every respect, as even this is bound to be selective, but it helps,

[13] *Op. cit.*

and furthermore it prevents the falsifying process of secondary elaboration. Moreover this writing down should be done without the co-operation of anybody else, as in this way suggestion is excluded.

INTERVIEWS

Being interviewed has become so familiar a facet of modern life that we tend to forget that interviews are not just a matter of questions being plied higgledy-piggledy, but conform to an underlying pattern. When we visit a doctor, it is essential that the meeting does not become a conversation. The physician has to find out certain things thoroughly, and in these days of long queues in the waiting room, quickly. Similarly when Richard Dimbleby interviews the Dame of Sark for the sake of so many million of television viewers, it is essential that his questions are framed with the intent of providing information to those that look on. And when a series of candidates are being surveyed for a job, there are a number of specific questions that have to be asked from each one of them. Plainly there has to be much study before the interview is enacted. Very often the interviewer has adopted a rule of thumb technique over a period of years. He knows exactly what questions to ask at what time. Other people have devoted more study to the problem and act accordingly. In either case, the knowledge that has been built up by psychologists over the years may be useful. It should be pointed out at once, however, that no amount of knowing *about* interviewing automatically makes a good interviewer. It only helps to avoid errors and save time, and makes one pay attention to details that might have been overlooked otherwise.

It would be perfectly possible to discuss particular kinds of interview—the clinical interview, the employment interview, and so on. We shall, however, discuss types of interviews according to their own intrinsic nature, which may or may not be relevant to a particular field, or number of fields. All interviews, of course, have as their common intention, the eliciting of information.

TYPES

There is a range of possible approaches in interviews, from the highly standardised type to the completely unstructured sort.

That is to say, the former kind is made of questions which are strictly determined in advance and the answers have a limited set of alternative responses, while the latter kind is characterised by an intentional non-determination. In this approach the interviewer is free to ask those questions which he deems appropriate at the time, and the respondent is not bound by fixed answers. The distinction can be made from the point of view of the type of question: a question can be "open" or "closed". A closed question permits a series of alternatives, yes or no, or yes, no or don't know. An open question has no indication as to the form of the answer. An unstructured interview with open questions does not mean that the interviewer does not interrogate without a framework. Even in the broadest kind of non-structured interview, as in the psycho-analytic session, the interviewer (analyst) keeps his questions to the point. Only he allows his patient—if the simile is permitted—a lot of rope with which to express his answers. We can look upon the interview as a net in which to catch some information. Sometimes the mesh is small, sometimes it is large, according to how we think the information is best caught. It is clear that in a therapeutic situation, where information is difficult to collect anyhow, the patient must be allowed a large amount of latitude in his answers. While in canvassing voters to learn if they will vote for this person or that person, all that is required is whether they will vote for the canvasser's candidate or not, or whether they do not know: three categories, yes, no, do not know. Intermediate between this type of interview and the completely non-structured kind is the "open-end" interview. The respondent is not bound to limited alternatives, he is allowed to frame his replies in any way he likes. The questions are predetermined, but the interviewer is allowed to probe further by asking such questions as "What makes you think so?" and "In what way do you mean?", questions which are non-directive and devised to find more about the attitude of the respondent.

Taking the above types of interviews as within the range of "standardised" to "unstandardised", the question might be asked as to which is preferable. The arguments in favour of each have been summarised as follows:[14]

"In favor of standardised interviews:

[14] Maccoby, E. E., and Maccoby, N. "The Interview: A Tool of Social Science". In Lindzey, G.: *Handbook of Social Psychology*. Vol. I. Addison-Wesley 1954.

(*a*) they incorporate a basic principle of measurement: that of making information comparable from case to case,

(*b*) they are more reliable,

(*c*) they minimise errors of question wording.

In favor of unstandardised interviews:

(*a*) they permit standardisation of *meanings* rather than of the more superficial aspects of the stimulus situation,

(*b*) they are more valid, in that they encourage more true-to-life replies,

(*c*) they are more flexible."

In social work, interviews adopt a somewhat intermediate position, although the varieties of work involved determine which kind is used. Later paragraphs will investigate more closely the role of interviews in social work.

THE INTERVIEWER

There was an anecdote current during the early years of the last war, when women were drafted to factories and hospitals, to the effect that a middle-aged lady was interviewed by a young girl as to the work to be chosen. When the applicant had turned down three suggestions by the girl at the labour exchange, the latter rather petulantly asked "Well, what *do* you want to do?" To which the forthright answer came: "Sit down all the day on my bottom, like you." Whether the story is apocryphal or not, it indicates that the nature of the interviewer has an effect on the issue. Clearly it is not intelligent policy to employ young girls to direct women of double their age to irksome and laborious jobs, or at least not unsympathetic young girls. Clearly it is false policy to employ Semitic interviewers on a survey concerning attitudes to Jews. Similarly class differences between interviewer and respondents may result in a loss of content.

Perception of the Interviewer. However it is not only the manner and appearance of the interviewer that mars the situation, as the *perception* of the interviewer by the respondent. Sheatsley[15] has endorsed this by saying that "The interviewer's manner and appearance can of course, alter the respondent's perception of

[15] Sheatsley, Paul B. "The Art of Interviewing and a Guide to Interviewer Selection and Training". In Jahoda, M., Deutsch, M. and Cook, S.: *Research Methods in Social Relations.* Part Two. Dryden Press 1951.

him, but there is an abundance of experimental evidence to prove that bias may result, under certain conditions, regardless of anything the interviewer may do to eliminate it. In one study, 50 per cent of a sample of non-Jewish respondents told non-Jewish interviewers that they thought Jews had too much influence in the business world, whereas only 22 per cent of an equivalent sample voiced that opinion to Jewish interviewers. . . . Such effects can occur easily no matter how conscientiously the interviewer attempts to be 'unbiassed'."

This, then, is a matter about which the interviewer himself can do little. It is to higher authorities, that select the interviewers, that this difficulty should be placed. The above examples concern the "Poll" type of interview, where an opinion is to be learned. The effect, however, may have a similar influence in the kind of interviews involving social workers. A health visitor, for example may exacerbate a busy housewife concerning the well-being of the children, not because the health visitor lacks tact or is officious, or any of these things; it is because the health visitor is a "Miss". And however knowledgeable the worker may be about children, it is the respondent's perception of her that matters, and because she is not a mother there may be the idea at the back of the housewife's mind to the effect that the interviewer does not know the personal problems concerning children.

Perception of the Interviewed. Besides the question of the perception of the interviewer, there is the perception of the respondent. However impartial interviewers may try to become, there could be cases where the latter is influenced by the person he is questioning. An interviewer is but human, and he has attitudes and opinions which may creep into his judgement. We shall have occasion in a moment to note the bias of interviewers; at this point attention can be drawn to the fact that in a more or less unstructured interview, the choice of further probing a question lies purely in the hands of the interviewer, and that he may feel inclined or disinclined to do this according to the nature of the person with whom he is in discourse. As the author from whose chapter on interviewing we have quoted has stated: "Thus, given the same 'No opinion' response from a wealthy businessman, in the one case, and from a Negro housewife in another, they may probe the former's reply, in the complete belief that an opinion *must* be lurking somewhere, whereas in the latter they will routinely accept it without probing and go on to the next question."

In most instances in social work, there is no question of specially selected interviewers nor of formal training of present workers. Interviews are just part and parcel of the other work. Therefore what has been said before and will be said about the nature of interviewers and the art of interviewing is presented as information from which the interested worker can learn, and is not intended to be applied directly. In social work, as in clinical situations, rapport with the client is an essential feature. The merits of paying attention to reliable features of interviewing should not interfere with the art of making the client feel "at home". Indeed, as we shall see when discussing techniques of interviewing, this is the primary advice.

Interviewer Bias. We have mentioned the manner and appearance of the interviewer as providing a bias. Just how much this bias can be is afforded by the study made by Katz[16] on the social status of interviewers in public opinion polls. The respondents in this case, amounting to about six hundred interviews in all, came from the poor quarter of Pittsburgh. Now there were two teams of interviewers, both with exactly the same set of instructions and questions, but the one was composed of white-collar workers and the other was composed of individuals from the working class. The result of the study showed that there were marked differences in the reports of the two teams. The middle-class white-collar interviewer, for example, found a "greater incidence of conservative attitudes among lower income groups than do interviewers recruited from the working class". There have been similar studies made with similar findings using the colour of the interviewer as the variable to be tested. In this example the bias arises from the perception by the respondent of his interviewer. It is to be expected that another type of bias will have as its source the attitude of the interviewer himself. Thus Cantril[17] made an investigation of a ballot to inquire into the opinions of Americans who favoured helping England or who held to the viewpoint that they should stay out of the war at all costs. The study was made in 1940.

[16] Katz, D. "Do interviewers bias poll results?" *Publ. Opin. Quart.* 1942, **6**, 248.
[17] Cantril, H. *Gauging Public Opinion.* Princeton Univ. Press, 1944.

Communication

Cantril found that interviewers (who had also filed their opinions) who themselves were for helping England managed to collect more votes for this viewpoint than for keeping out of the war. While in the case of interviewers who favoured the last opinion, the role was reversed, they collected more opinions for staying out of the war.

A projection or suggestion of the attitude of an interviewer may be quite open and intentional. It can also be quite unintentional; that is to say it can be quite unconscious on the part of the interviewer, who puts over his biases without meaning to. In an unstandardised interview, or one where the choice of questions is slightly manoeuverable, there need only be a casual turn of phrase to allow the interviewer's own attitude to make its way felt. Unless the latter is sufficiently alive to this factor, the interview will be marred by "interviewer effect".

INTERVIEWS IN SOCIAL WORK

In many ways the type of interview necessary in social work is peculiar to its own discipline, and it is not so easy to translate principles and advice from other fields to it. Nevertheless there are points of accord between them which will become apparent as we note the factors and principles in social work interviewing.

Relief of Anxiety. As might be expected in this type of work, one of the first principles is to put the client at ease. In social case work and child guidance fields the investigators have placed this first in importance.[18] In a child guidance study it was found that the first task in the interview was to release anxiety, both about the child and about the function of the clinic itself. It was recommended that "A brief statement about the real function of the clinic will help to reduce first tensions; and most parents will relax into comparative calm when told that masturbation is common among children, or that a child charged with larceny is not necessarily a potential criminal." Anxiety also is the key-note arising from a study of interviews with relatives of patients in a mental hospital.[19] In the first place there were fears and anxieties

[18] Colcord, J. C. "A study of the technique of the Social Case Work interview". *Social Forces* 1929, 7, 519. Castle, R. M. and Williams, J. J. B. "Notes on initial interviews in Child Guidance". *Brit. J. Psychiatric Social Work*, 1947, September, 75.
[19] Goodale, E. "Intake interviews with relatives of psychotic patients". *Smith College Studies in Social Work*. 1944–5, 15, 15.

140

about the hospital; then there were anxieties about the patient which were largely imaginary and subjective; and there were guilt feelings based upon the fear of disapproval of their handling of the patient-relative.

The Wording of Questions. The phrasing of questions, as we have already noted under the subject of Testimony, is a difficult art. But apart from the point of imputing responses, there is the important matter of getting the client to talk in the first place. From the standpoint of hospital interviewing Snelling[20] recommends caution in this respect. "The wording of questions demands special care, as the negative question is a trap for the nervous patient. 'You aren't worried about your job, are you?' invites the answer 'No', and he may say 'No' even when he wishes to say 'Yes'. With the direct question a moment's preliminary thought can prevent an impasse. 'Have you relatives to look after the children while you come into hospital?' may bring a flat 'No', and then both patient and social worker face a blank wall; but the question 'What relatives have you?' may produce the reply, 'I have a sister in Wales, but I can't afford to pay her fare to come here', and the wall is then less blank."

The Number of Interviews. A particular question which is very relevant to the arrival of a new client is how many interviews will he attend. It may be useful to be able to differentiate the one-interview client from the "more than one interview" person. Blenkner[21] has made a study concerning this and found four factors to be operative. The first is the actual problem for which the client sought assistance. Problems of a primary psychological or inter-personal nature resulted in a number of interviews as distinguished from the case where the problems arose from some other area. The second factor concerns the client's response to the worker's suggestion for solution of the basic problem. If it was found that the response of the client to this was non-committal or downright rejecting, then the client seldom came for another meeting. The client's conception of the role of the worker at the beginning of the

[20] Snelling, Jean. "Some notes on hospital interviewing". *Social Work* 1947, *4*, 10.
[21] Blenkner, Margaret, "Predictive Factors in the Initial Interview in Family Casework". *Social Service Review* 1954, *28*, 65.

interview was an important third factor. If the worker was regarded as a counsellor and not merely as the avenue to a service, then this made for follow-up interviews. Continuing on from this (the fourth factor), if the worker was accepted by the client as a counsellor at the *end* of the interview, then this too made for a number of interviews. The conclusions in this study were drawn from a sample of 360 persons, in family casework, in the United States. It is not expected that there would be very great divergences in the British Isles or elsewhere, but this may be a matter where cultural differences have some influence, and further research is necessary. Again the type of agency may be another persuasive variable, and this too needs investigation.

The above quotations surveying in part the wide variance of types of interviews, the problems arising in them, and the value of prognosis, in social work, draw attention to the individual nature of interviews in social work. Because of this feature "standardised" interviews are likely to be the exception rather than the rule in social work, although this does not preclude a systematic approach by the interviewer.

TECHNIQUES

It is sufficiently apparent that the first step in a social work interview is the task of putting the client at his ease and establishing rapport. This is perhaps so obvious that it does not need reiteration. Only, in the desire to extract relevant information and to avoid a delay in time, these initial considerations are sometimes forgotten. Now in stating techniques for the interview, it is only possible to provide generalisations; the variety of clients and situations in the interviews germane to social work make particular applications too many to enumerate. Furthermore it is to be expected that individual workers have evolved their own form of enquiry after years of experience, which within the limits of their type of work, appears to be rewarding. In furnishing generalisations, we shall refer to the conclusions of Oldfield's book, *The Psychology of The Interview*,[22] which is recommended for further study. Oldfield first makes the comment that the interview should not be regarded as something on its own, but the application of skills that are familiar aspects of social life, that is the use of conversation and expression and other features that are involved

[22] Oldfield, R. C. *The Psychology of the Interview*. Methuen 1941.

in the daily transaction of living with other people. Oldfield emphasises strongly the concept of "attitude" as being the cornerstone of the interview. As he puts it, "it (conversation) is, first and foremost, a game played directly in terms of *attitudes*; and the use to which it is put in the interview can be properly appreciated only in these terms." The purpose of this volume, as the author himself says, was not to end up with a number of practical suggestions, but to inculcate "a spirit of inquiry among interviewers." However he does make a number of suggestions, and it is deemed worthwhile to quote these. Oldfield lists seven in all. First he advises would-be interviewers to cultivate the art of human relations in general, and not necessarily to study those people with whom they come into professional contact. Following on from this it is recommended that a knowledge of human nature should be developed, by any means. The third suggestion, axiomatic to students of social work, is that the interviewer should look to his own changes in attitudes, and cultivate an introspective habit of mind. With regard to the actual interview situation, Oldfield maintains that the objective of it must always be kept in mind, and not allowed to degenerate into a number of unconnected observations. He stresses, too, that the interviewer should think and act in terms of attitudes, " 'Never mind *what* the candidate says: notice the *way* he says it', 'Don't try to make the *correct remark*: think instead of the *appropriate attitude* to take up, and a suitable form of words will be forthcoming.' " The suggestions end up with a caution of the use of ordinary words.

The above practical hints were not purported for social work interviews, but the suggestions are of a degree of generalisation to allow for this application. What remains to be said is this: there is no formal training for interviews in social work, and there is always a gap between the written advice and the execution of it. Unintelligent application of intelligent practical suggestions is probably worse than if advice had not been followed in the first place. That is why there can never be any fixed rules of interviews of the unstandardised type. There can only be a few guiding principles (of the kind which Oldfield has put forward); and a few blatant mistakes which are often made by people new to interviewing can be pointed out. Anything more than this can only be amplified by the interviewer in his or her unique situation.

NON-VERBAL COMMUNICATION

The type of communication we have been discussing up to now has been explicitly verbal. Anyone who has experienced the initial stages of a flirtation is well aware that there are other than verbal methods of imparting and receiving information. A great deal of information is imparted through gestures in daily inter-course. Only as these are performed along with the spoken word, their message is often lost. By gestures is meant not only move-ments of arms and legs, but also facial expression. At a rather more subtle level muscular tensions play their role. How relevant this may be is suggested by the references in the Old Testament to the Israelites as a stiff-necked people. The expression is still with us. Then there is the exclusively interpersonal mechanism, which can be regarded from the point of view of communication, whereby emotional attitudes are transferred between people. All these non-verbal modes of communication may not be prominent, are in fact in the background of interpersonal relationships, yet nevertheless are important.

EMOTIONAL EXPRESSION

We learn that a person is angry, afraid, happy, sad, disgusted or sulky from the expressions of his face and possibly the actions of other parts of his body in addition. A speaker need not be verbally informed by one of his audience that his discourse is boring; it is, as we say, "written all over" his listener's face. Nevertheless, although in many situations an emotion can be accurately judged, experi-mental researches have shown that this is not always the case.

Recognition of Emotions. The procedure in the experimental study of judgement of emotions is quite simply to present a picture showing an expression of some emotion to a group of subjects and ask them to label it. When this is done, without any guiding information at all, responses can be very varied. To quote a typical study:[23] motion pictures were taken of the emotional expressions of infants aroused by hunger, pain, being dropped and restraint. These were shown to medical students and nurses, who were of course well accustomed to the reactions of babies. Results

[23] Sherman, M. "The Differentiation of Emotional Responses in Infants". *J. Comp. Psychol.* 1927, 7, 265 and 335.

showed that accuracy of the emotion portrayed was little better than guess work. Only when the judges were given information of the stimulus to the emotion—being dropped for example—was there better accuracy. An earlier study[24] using photographs of a whole series of emotions had much the same result. The greatest disagreement was about the emotional expressions representing anger, fear and suspicion, hate and rage. The least disagreement occurred with the expressions of disgust and sneering.

These two studies, the first using spontaneous reactions of infants, the second employing intentional expressions of an actress, would seem to suggest that the interpretation of an emotion by facial expression alone is very inaccurate. However Woodworth[25] has demonstrated that this is not necessarily the case. Early studies had not taken into account the measure of the degree of error. As Woodworth puts it, "We need to scrutinise the judgements, asking *how far wrong* they are. We need a scale, rough though it may be, for measuring the error." Accordingly, Woodworth arranged the type of emotions that had been used in the previously mentioned second study in a single series with similar emotions adjoining. This order would allow for a near mistake in categorising. For example, by placing happiness next to love at one end of the scale, and disgust next to contempt at the other end of the same scale, the fact that the emotional expression depicting love would be mistaken for happiness, could be contrasted with the fact that it was mistaken for contempt. When a scale like this is adapted to methods of recognising emotional expressions, the judgements are fairly accurate. In Woodworth's own study, the pose for fear was recognised *as* fear by sixty-six per cent of the subjects, as anger by nineteen per cent, as suffering and surprise by about five per cent. Thus the finding that recognition of the emotions is haphazard has to be modified.

The Influence of Cultures. We tend to conjoin a particular gesture with a particular meaning; raising of the eyebrows indicates with us interrogation or incredulity. In the case of George Robey it indicated mirth. The context of an expression is related to the conventional signs of a community. One becomes so accustomed

[24] Feleky, A. M. "The Expression of the Emotions". *Psychol. Review* 1914, *21*, 33.
[25] Woodworth, R. S. *Experimental Psychology*. Holt, 1938, "The student is referred to Chapter XI "Expression of the Emotions" for further study.

to the conventions of one's own society, with its habitual modes of expression, that a study of the influence of different cultures on emotional expression is often surprising. The following list of expressions, gestures and habits of different cultures with their appropriate meanings, shows the wide variety of interpretations given to a similar act.[26] Hissing in our culture is a rude way of disapproval; in Japan on the other hand it is a form of politeness to social superiors. The Basuto actually applaud by hissing. Spitting in our culture is hardly a sign of affection, yet among the Masai of East Africa it means exactly that. We stand up in the presence of superiors; in Polynesia, the Fijians and the Tongans sit down. "The Toda of South India raise the open right hand to the face, with the thumb on the bridge of the nose, to express respect; a gesture almost identical among Europeans is an obscene expression of extreme disrespect. Placing to the tip of the nose the projecting knuckle of the right forefinger bent at the second joint was among the Maori of New Zealand a sign of friendship and often of protection; but in eighteenth-century England the placing of the same forefinger to the right side of the nose expressed dubiousness about the intelligence and sanity of the speaker—much as does the twentieth-century clockwise motion of the forefinger above the right hemisphere of the head". The list could be extended; it is enough to have shown a few examples to illustrate the fact that the interpretation of an emotional expression depends very much upon the social context in which it has been acquired.

TRANSFERENCE

The phenomenon of transference arose from the technique of psycho-analysis,[27] but there is little doubt that it is not peculiar to the relationship between the analyst and his patient. It probably exists, in varying degrees, whenever there is emotional communication between people, but particularly in relationships such as those between doctor and patient, teacher and pupil, and social worker and client. The meaning of the term alludes to the fact that in the relationship between the analyst and his patient, the

[26] Quoted from LaBarre, W. "The cultural basis of emotions and gestures". *J. Personality* 1947, *16*, 49.

[27] See the Chapter on it in Freud, S. *Introductory Lectures on Psycho-Analysis*. Allen & Unwin, 1922, Chapter 27.

latter tends to transfer to the physician affections and thoughts which, at an earlier period of his life, had been associated with somebody else, particularly with parental figures. Thus the patient tends to regard the analyst as a sort of father and to repeat a class of behaviour with him which was similar to the behaviour shown at a much earlier stage of his life. This may exhibit itself in a number of ways. One of the most important ways was that of sexual interest. Female patients displayed an interest in the analyst which could only be described as erotic. Male patients displayed negative transference, that is they tended to resent the authority of the physician and become hostile to him. This was interpreted in classical psycho-analysis as being connected with the erotic attachments which boys have to their mothers and girls to their fathers. (For a description of these complexes see the following Chapter.) Girls who were in love with their fathers now repeated this disposition with their new father figures; boys who were in love with their mother and resented their father, carried over this attitude to the relations with the analyst. It is part of the psycho-analytic therapy to take the fact of transference into account. It must be recognised, interpreted and "won through". It is no part of our intention here to describe the practical technique of psycho-analysis; it is to draw attention to a form of interpersonal communication that is particularly subtle and difficult to assess. It is a phenomenon that is particularly relevant in casework. As one writer has stressed:[28] "some degree of transference is always present, and it can reach considerable intensity in a casework situation, *whether client and worker recognise it or not*. In fact we are coming to realise that one reason why it is important for every caseworker to be able to recognise transference phenomena is that it is necessary to recognise them in order to be able to modify and control them."

While it was the view of Freud that transference was the reactivation of events in the past, the view has been put forward[29] that it can be divorced from this interpretation of infantile origins, and can be recognised as a form of present disturbance in human relationships that takes place between analyst and patient as well as elsewhere. Transference it to be understood in the light

[28] Irvine, E. E. "Transference and Reality in the Casework Relationship". *Brit. J. Psychiatric Social Work* 1956, *3*, No. 4 p. 15.
[29] By Horney, Karen. *New Ways in Psycho-Analysis*. Kegan Paul 1939.

of the whole actual structure of the personality at the present time and not necessarily to be related to factors in childhood. Other viewpoints[30] have stressed the reaction to authority as being a vital element in interpreting the phenomenon. Whatever interpretation is given, the fact is not disavowed, and it remains undoubtedly a significant factor in interpersonal communication.

[30] For example, H. S. Sullivan and E. Fromm.

VI

PERSONALITY

THERE are some terms in Psychology which possess a multiplicity of definitions. "Set" is one such term, "attitude" is another, and the subject of this last chapter is clearly another. Allport, writing in 1937,[1] listed forty-eight definitions used in the past, and then provided the forty-ninth and fiftieth. Definitions of Personality range from omnibus interpretations to interpretations in a framework of adjustment or integration. And they sometimes differ according to the slant of a school of thought. If one confined the study of personality to the single task of taxonomy, the discipline would become far more complex than indeed it is already. Enumeration of the varieties of individuals, in the psychological sense, could there even be found a fundamental basis of classification, would overshadow the efforts of the biologists of the seventeenth and eighteenth centuries—men such as Ray and Cuvier and the Swede, Linneaus, who attempted to classify the world of plants and animals. So it is not surprising that many psychologists have eschewed this approach, and merely given a working definition, as Allport does for his book. In this volume, although for the sake of exposition, we shall approach the subject from different viewpoints, from the biological position, from the social standpoint and so on, if it helps the reader to have *some* kind of definition, then we can do no better than in fact to use Allport's working definition, which is: "Personality is the dynamic organisation within the individual of those psychophysical systems that determine his unique adjustments to his environment."

[1] Allport, G. W. *Personality: A Psychological Interpretation.* Constable 1937.

Analysis and Synthesis. Both analysis and synthesis when applied to the study of personality have limitations. Analysis takes up various approaches, renders the complex material easier to understand, but loses the essential ingredient, namely the individual that is analysed. After tearing a person into his biological and social components, it is difficult to say as Mark Antony said of Brutus, "This was a man", unless we apply it cynically with the emphasis on the past tense of the auxiliary verb. Synthesis, on the other hand, may keep the essential but leaves the myriad-like aspect untouched; it is at once too embracing and too narrow. The distinction in approach has been called the "nomothetic" as against the "idiographic" way of describing personality. The emphasis in the nomothetic approach is to analyse the components of personality common to all individuals, while in the ideographic approach the insistence is upon personality as a unique configuration which cannot be analysed into its component parts.

DEFINITIONS

In this Chapter we shall adopt an analysis of personality by tracing the various determinants of it—biological, psychological and social. The discussion of these will occupy the next three sections. In this section it is necessary to provide both working definitions of some of the aspects of personality discussed, and to describe some of the methods of measuring personality.

Temperament and Character. These two terms have often been used as synonymous with personality itself, but we shall define them as aspects of it. Temperament has been regarded as the constellation of the emotional and impulsive aspects in experience, which are characteristic of an individual. We describe people as being cheerful, gloomy, excitable, calm, optimistic and pessimistic and so forth, which are all adjectives designating temperament. The Greeks devised a scheme, a classification of temperament, based on the notion of humours or fluids of the body, which divided emotional dispositions into four groups, which they called sanguine, phlegmatic, choleric and melancholic. Today the theory is discredited, but the fact that emotions are bound up with the internal workings of our bodies is very true. A resumé of the modern conception of this aspect will be given in the next section.

Broadly speaking, while personality is considered to be the sum total of the physical, mental, moral and social qualities of a person, character pertains to integration of these tendencies from the standpoint of a social or ethical criterion. When we say that X is a "bad character" we are saying that certain aspects of this person's personality are not in accordance with the type of behaviour which in our society we designate as "good". Besides this, the term "character traits" is often used to describe the relatively enduring features of personality, the ones which as we say are "characteristic" of a person.

Traits and Types. As suggested in the last few lines, a trait is a characteristic feature of personality. It cuts across the classification of temperament and character, as both these aspects of personality are made up by traits. "Cheerful" is a trait and so is "honesty". A personality is made up of scores of traits. Obviously, from the point of view of evaluation, it would be simpler if we could find some way of reducing this large number to a smaller quantity. A method of doing this is *factor analysis*,[2] whereby traits are clustered into groups and correlated with one another. Those traits that correlate well with one another are abridged under one basic trait or factor. In this way a number of traits can be reduced to a few common factors.

A type is generally an example of an extreme feature in personality, common to a class of individuals. Jung's classification of introvert and extrovert is an example. An introvert is a person who turns his interest inwards to his own thoughts and feelings, while an extrovert characteristically is more interested in the world about him. But these are the extreme cases. Most people are a mixture of introvert and extrovert. If we think of types as being in separate compartments, its use as a way of defining personalities is misleading. Rather we should think of types as being selected points on a continuum; in the above case both would be the extreme points, at either end. When we discuss constitutional types in the next section, the advantage of defining along a continuous scale will be recognised.

---

[2] A proper description of factor analysis with its mathematical basis is beyond the scope of this book. In regard to its application to the study of personality, the student is referred to Eysenck, H. J. *Dimensions of Personality.* Kegan Paul 1947.

THE MEASUREMENT OF PERSONALITY

The following four methods of testing personality will be reviewed: Rating scales, Questionnaires and Inventories, Situational Tests, and Projective methods.

Rating Scales. There are several types of rating scales. One of the most common is simply to make judgement on a number of traits by indicating an assessment along a prepared list of descriptions. For example if a person was being judged for honesty, a five or seven point scale ranging from extreme honesty to extreme dishonesty, with the intermediate steps in between, would be given to somebody to indicate their rating by checking at the appropriate place. The scale might run, if there were only five points: Very honest, honest, half honest and half dishonest, dishonest, very dishonest; all that the judge has to do is to place a tick at one of these points. Descriptions need not be given, and the quantitative scale can be given alone, the higher the number indicating more of the trait judged. The advantage of rating scales is that intermediate steps are allowed for; to judge a man as *either* honest *or* dishonest is likely to be too sweeping an assertion. It also fails to differentiate different people accurately enough. Also two or three or more judges can use the same scale on one person and their assessment can be pooled. Finally it is a relatively easy method to apply.

Questionnaires and Inventories. The simplest form of questionnaire merely consists of a number of statements to which a person must answer "yes" or "no". Sometimes a third category "don't know" is included. Or the statements may be in the form to which answers of "true" and "false" are the appropriate responses. The questionnaire approach has wide applicability. It can be used to find out people's interests, their attitudes towards religion and politics, their emotional maladjustments, and their positions on any selected continuum of traits such as ascendancy-submission. The advantage of questionnaires and inventories is that they can be easily applied and if properly constructed can cull valuable information about a person. The disadvantages are that many questionnaires are easy to "fool"; that is to say, if a person knows what the series of questions is after, he can frame his answers according to what impression he wishes to give. Also many questionnaires, by their set number of possible answers, impose artificial responses. A solution to the first difficulty is overcome by incorporating in the whole range of questions some which are specially designed to test lying. The second difficulty is met by including rating scales attached to each question.[3]

Situational Tests. Instead of attempting to discover the personality of a person by paper and pencil methods, there is the possibility of testing for a selected trait by miniature real life situations. One type of this kind of test was devised in the Character Education Inquiry carried out by Hartshorne and May.[4] Here children were tested for a number of characteristics, such as honesty, truthfulness, self-control and generosity. A typical situational test was involved in the studies on cheating. The children were given pencil and paper problems to solve, which were then collected and a duplicate set of each child's answers made. Afterwards the original papers were then returned to the children with a key for self-scoring. It could then be seen, by comparing the original and the duplicate, whether the child had cheated in scoring his own paper by altering his responses. In other words the situation was deliberately contrived to allow for any sign of dishonesty to manifest.

Projective Methods. The principle in projection tests is to give an individual a series of pictures or statements which are deliberately open to all kinds of interpretations. In this way the subject is said to reveal his innermost needs, desires and attitudes, which would not be possible by a direct approach. The best known of these methods is the Rorschach ink blot test. Ten standard patterns of ink blots are given one at a time to a subject, who is simply asked to report what he sees or what he thinks the ink blots represent. The patterns are all bilaterally symmetrical, some are in black and white, others are in colour. Responses are measured according to

[3] This is only a sketch. Consult, for a full exposition, Jahoda, Deutsch and Cook. *Research Methods in Social Relations*, Part I, Chapter 6 especially.

[4] Hartshorne, H., and May, M. *Studies in the Nature of Character* Vol. I *Studies in Deceit*, MacMillan 1928; Vol. II (with Maller, J. B.) *Studies in Service and Self-Control*, MacMillan 1929; Vol. III (with Shuttleworth, F. K.), *Studies in the Organisation of Character* MacMillan 1930.

such factors as the part of the blot to which the subject makes his observation, or whether he regards the pattern as a whole or chooses some small detail. The form, colour and shading observed are further factors to be assessed, and whether movement is perceived. The content of the patterns suggest a range of perceptions of human figures to animals and plants, from anatomical diagrams to landscapes, and from maps to food. The scoring of this test is very complex. There are many possible responses which are given interpretations. Thus seeing humans in movement is regarded as an indication of fantasy living, reaction to the whole figure is assessed as conceptual thinking, responses determined primarily by colour, with form contributing are interpreted as an unstable emotional reaction.[5]

The drawback of the Rorschach test is that there is a poor standardisation of the interpretations of the responses. Judgements of personality from this device are prone to different subjective impressions by the person that uses it. When it is used by an experienced clinician along with other methods of measuring personality it has been found very useful in establishing clues to diagnosis.

Another type of projective method consists of giving a person incomplete sentences which he has to finish. For example the opening words may be "What annoys me . . ." "My greatest fear . . .", "Other people . . .", "I am best when . . .", "My greatest worry is . . .". The subject is then instructed to complete these sentences in order to express his real feelings. The rationale of the test, similar to all projective methods, is that a subject will reflect his own desires, fears and attitudes in the completed sentence.

The chief advantage of projective techniques is that they make available information about a person which is not readily accessible by other means, as the purpose of the test is disguised from the subject. He is more likely to reveal his secret wishes and fears in this way than by being directly probed. The disadvantages lie with the difficulties of standardisation, as discussed above.[6]

[5] For a concise description of the Rorschach see the Chapters by S. J. Beck and R. L. Munroe in Weider, A. *Contributions towards Medical Psychology* Vol. II. Ronald Press 1953.
[6] For a discussion of the merits and demerits of projective methods in general, see Anastasi, A. *Psychological Testing* Chapter 22. MacMillan 1954.

BIOLOGICAL ASPECTS

The organism operates in an integrative manner, and the various parts of which it is compounded are interdependent, so that one might justly state, if one looks upon personality as a configuration of the total response of the organism, that every part of the latter enters into what we call personality. Although this may be true, nevertheless there are some parts of the body which are relatively more important for personality manifestations, and we will proceed to discuss these.

THE ENDOCRINE SYSTEM

There are two main divisions of glands in the body, the duct glands and the ductless glands. The latter division differs from the former in that their secretions or hormones pass directly into the blood or lymph instead of into ducts and then excreted. Hence the ductless glands are also called the glands of internal secretion or the endocrine system, and it is this system which is important for the study of personality.

The endocrines represent an interlocking system on their own, as each gland has repercussions upon another, and if one over-secretes or under-secretes the whole system is thrown out of balance. Besides this it is integrated with the nervous system in such a way that the two are combined into a larger system. Abstracting the one from the other is necessary for exposition, but the integrative action of the nervous system must be kept in mind throughout.

Pituitary. Situated at the base of the brain, often called the "master-gland", is the Pituitary. It is composed of three parts, the posterior lobe, the anterior, and the segment that lies between. The first and the last need not concern us much in the discussion of personality, as the secretions produced are connected with the output of urine, the stimulation and contraction of blood vessels and the like. There is one hormone secreted by the posterior pituitary, however, which is of practical use; this is *pituitrin* which is employed clinically for increasing the tone of the muscles of the uterus in childbirth. It is the anterior pituitary that is of most importance for our subject, as this part has several hormones, which influence strongly the external behaviour of the organism.

Some of these hormones are related to growth and development. *Phyone* is the name given to the growth hormone of the anterior pituitary. If there is an abnormal increase of it during childhood there results an acceleration of the growth of the skeletal musculature, especially the long bones. The end result of this is gigantism. There is a variant of this when excessive secretion takes place not before growth has been completed, as in gigantism, but afterwards, when the condition known as acromegaly develops in which the bones of the face and the extremities of the body appear thickened. The reverse of over-secretion, that is when there is a retardation of the growth hormone during childhood, results in dwarfism. Another important secretion of the anterior pituitary is connected with sexual development. What has been termed the *gonadtropic* hormone stimulates the sexual glands and leads to their early development. It is possible, by injection of this hormone, to artificially start off the oestrus cycle in baby rats prematurely. There is a marked interrelation between the anterior pituitary and the sex glands. Not only does the pituitary "trigger-off" the action of the sex glands—the "motor of the gonads" as it has been paraphrased—but there is a reverse action. Oestrone (see below) in the blood acts on the pituitary and stops secretion of the gonadtropic hormone. It is interesting also to note that light controls the pituitary gland and hence the gonads. If pigeons are hooded, then eggs are delayed. Abnormal secretion of this hormone can lead to either precocious development of sexual characteristics, or renders the individual sexually immature, according to whether there is an over or under secretion. Again if the anterior pituitary is removed entirely puberty does not occur. The growth and the "sexual" secretions are not the sole hormones of this part of the pituitary, but as the other secretions are intimately connected with the functioning of the remaining endocrine organs, we will leave discussion of them until the latter have been reviewed.

Thyroid. The thyroid gland, situated as two lobes either side of the wind-pipe, is concerned with the regulation of the physical and chemical changes that go on continuously in the body, that is to say with metabolism. The hormone in this case is *thyroxin.* Again abnormal developments can occur. Cretinism, the term given to stunted physical and mental development, is due to an under-activity of this hormone in children. In adults if the thyroid becomes atrophied, then there is a noted obesity in the body with a concomitant sluggish behaviour, a condition known as myxoedema. On the other hand over-secretion gives rise to various kinds of nervous symptoms. One species of goitre, distinguished by nervousness, insomnia, and by protruding eyes, is caused by an enlarged thyroid.

Parathyroids. Situated close to the thyroid glands, similar in name but not in function, are the parathyroids, consisting of four small bodies. Their main action is to regulate the metabolism of calcium and phosphorus in the body. The parathyroids are related to behaviour in that nerve cells are unduly excited if calcium metabolism is reduced; hence some kinds of irritability may be due to a deficiency in their operation.

Liver. The liver is the fourth of the endocrine organs to be considered. As is well known it stores excess sugar as glycogen. When it is demanded it returns this to the blood stream. It also has other important physiological properties, which we need not consider here. The storing of excess sugar is important for occasions when there is required more energy, as in physical work or in a strenuous game involving constant use of the musculature, or alternatively in emotional situations.

Pancreas. In this storing of sugar, the liver is very much related to the working of the pancreas, in particular the small masses of cells called the islands of Langerhans. The function of these cells is to produce insulin (the deficiency of which causes diabetes), which increases the allowance of the passage of blood sugar through the walls of the cell. When insulin secretion is under the normal amount, as in diabetes, the blood sugar level increases, due to the fact that sugar cannot get into the liver where it would be stored, or into the body tissues where it would be used up. The pancreas and the liver thus are an interdependent pair of organs in relation to the storing of sugar, and the use of it by the organism.

Adrenals. The adrenal glands are the next consideration. They are situated on the kidney, with two distinct parts, the internal structure known as the medulla, and the outer covering called the cortex. (In parenthesis, it is useful to remember in order not to become hopelessly confused with these terms, that the word "medulla" is merely the Latin for marrow, and word "cortex" is the Latin for bark.) The adrenal medulla secretes the hormone *adrenalin*, which is very important in emotional reaction. Adrenalin has the effect of distributing the level of the blood sugar, and allows the passage of more fuel and oxygen to the musculature involved in emergency reactions. The cortex has various functions. It is related to the level of salt in the organisms. The secretion called *cortin* performs this latter function. It is also related to sexual characteristics. An over-allowance of cortin in the blood creates secondary male characteristics in girls, and abnormal virility in boys.

The Pituitary and Adrenal. There is an important relationship between the adrenal cortex and the pituitary. When the body is exposed to conditions of stress[7] and most parts of the body are marked by degenerative changes, there is one structure which appears to thrive in such conditions. This is the adrenal cortex. When the adrenal cortex is extirpated in experimental animals, and the animal is then put under conditions of stress, there is no "fighting response" exhibited by the organism. Conversely, if such an animal is artificially injected by a preparation from one of the hormones in the cortex, the "fighting instinct" is regained. Now it has been discovered that extirpation of the pituitary prevents this adrenal response, and the mechanism at work here is the hormone known as the *adreno-corticotropic* hormone, A.C.T.H. for short. As removal of the anterior pituitary prevents the characteristic response of the adrenals, it is concluded that stress stimulates the cortex through the pituitary via A.C.T.H.

Gonads. The sex glands, or gonads, including the ovaries in the female and the testes in the male, secrete a number of hormones, besides producing ova and sperms, the agencies of reproduction. We shall expound here not this latter important aspect, but the endocrine function of them, the secretions that produce the main differences between male and female. The formation of the sexual

[7] The Finding of Hans Selye reported in many publications. See "The general-adaptation-syndrome in its relationships to neurology, psychology and psychopathology". Chapter 11 of Weider, A. (ed.) *Contributions Toward Medical Psychology*, Vol. I. Ronald Press 1953.

hormones and the interrelation of them with other parts of the body is far more complicated than the following exposition will allow. The predominant sexual hormones are the *oestrogens* in the female and the *androgens* in the male. Of the oestrogens, the chief hormone is *oestrone*, which brings on heat. Another hormone, *progesterone*, is essential for the early stages of growth of the embryo. Of the male hormones, or androgens, *testosterone* is the most well known; it is responsible for the secondary male characteristics. It is not to be thought that these hormones are exclusive to either sex. It is only the predominant amount of oestrogens that are found in the female and the predominant amount of androgens found in the male. There are a small amount of female hormones in males and male hormones in females. In fact in rare cases of male homosexuals the proportion has been found to have been abnormal, and clinical redress can be made by proper injections of the appropriate hormones. Furthermore it is not only the gonads that contain the sex hormones; the adrenal cortex also contains them. In fact the pituitary, adrenal cortex and the gonads form a functional triad in relation to sexual characteristics.

There are two remaining glands which have not yet been discussed. These are the thymus gland and the pineal. Very little is known about either; there are no known active secretions.

Interdependence. Much has already been said about the interrelations of some of these endocrine glands. It is necessary to stress this interdependence again. Together they present a homeostatic mechanism of some of the most important chemical constituents of the organism. They play an important part in the behaviour of the individual. Part to part they act as a system of balance and counter-balance. As Freeman[8] has exemplified: "The pancreas opposes the action of the pituitary, and the adrenals oppose the action of the pancreas. Development of the sex glands is held in check by the pineal, thymus, the adrenals, the thyroid, and the pituitary, and is advanced by other substances from some of these same glands. If the thyroid becomes hyperactive, the rate of metabolism is raised and other glands become overactive as well. A hyperactive thyroid may be due either to excessive adrenal action or to lowered pituitary action. When the ovaries

[8] Freeman, G. L. *Physiological Psychology.* Van Nostrand Co. 1948.

atrophy at the menopause, the thyroid is left without its usual counterbalancing hormone, and the hyperactive thyroid condition which develops stimulates a compensatory overactivity of the adrenals with resulting nervous symptoms."

ENZYMES AND VITAMINS

Hormones, enzymes and vitamins are chemical agents that assist in regulating the chemical factory that is the organism. Of these we have already discussed the first. We now turn to enzymes and vitamins, which both influence behaviour. An enzyme is an organic substance which causes speedy complex transformations of chemical elements in the organism. The best known example of this occurs in digestion. The food that enters the mouth is broken down into simpler chemical elements by the action of enzymes, so that the energy latent in foodstuffs is employed for the various activities of the body. And the enzymes perform this important breaking-down activity without themselves entering into the reaction: a process called *catalysis*. Enzymes are thus *catalysts*. The role of enzymes in behaviour is one that is still very much under research, and the complexity of it is immense. Although much is still hypothetical, there is reason to suggest that some types of mental illness are caused by the maladjustment of some enzyme systems in the brain.[9]

Vitamins differ from both hormones and enzymes in that they are not produced by the body. They are organic substances which occur in various kinds of food. As is well known they are essential for a normal diet. Personality effects can be artificially induced by restriction of certain vitamins. Psychoneuroses can be induced for example by the experimental restriction of a vitamin called *thiamine*. In fact there has been coined a new term—avitaminosis—as a rubric for the effect of vitamins on behaviour.[10] As with the role of enzymes, however, further research will cast light for their full part in personality.

BRAIN STRUCTURE

It is not possible to delve here into all the functions of the brain, and the operations of each part. We are discussing personality,

[9] See Pope, A. "Enzymatic Changes in Mental Diseases" in *The Biology of Mental Health and Disease*. Hoeber 1952.

[10] Wilder, R. M. "Experimental Induction of Psychoneuroses through restriction of intake of Thiamine". In *Biology of Mental Health and Disease*.

and we shall have to limit the exposition to this subject. It is necessary though to sketch in the main parts of the brain and their functions in order to provide a framework for what follows. It will be the very simplest of outlines. The reader is advised to turn to an elementary volume of anatomy and physiology for further reference.

Division of the Brain. The entire brain can be divided into three parts, the cerebral hemispheres, the midbrain and the hindbrain. Proceeding in the reverse order, the hindbrain contains parts related to vital centres controlling circulation and respiration. It also contains that large structure under the back of the head called the *cerebellum*, which has to do with the maintenance of equilibrium and the integration of voluntary movements. Recent research has shown that the cerebellum has much in common with the cerebral hemispheres.

The midbrain embraces parts that co-ordinate reflexes of eye and posture. The fact that a falling cat always lands upon its feet is due to a complex system of reflexes which always sees that the animal is right side up in relation to the external world.

The cerebral hemispheres are our main concern. In man the evolutionary older parts of the two spheres are covered, or to be more exact are convoluted, by the grey tissue known as the *cerebral cortex*, the region most lately evolved and dealing with the manifold activities common to the higher animals. Underneath the cortex lie older centres for movements, and in particular an area known as the *diencephalon*. One part of this, the *thalamus*, is a most important relay centre for the transmission of messages from lower levels of the central nervous system to the cerebral cortex. In lower animals the thalamus is the highest sensory centre. In the diencephalon also is the *hypothalamus*, which contains the higher co-ordinating centres for the control of the autonomic system. It has much to do with the functioning of emotions.

The Cerebral Cortex. There are four lobes to the cerebral cortex, the frontal, temporal, parietal and occipital. It is convenient to classify the functions according to whether they are sensory or motor, that is whether the different areas of the cortex are terminal areas for impulses arising from events in the external world through the senses or from impulses within the body itself, or whether the various areas have to do with voluntary movement of the body.

The sensory areas are located in three of the lobes: parietal, temporal and occipital. Centres concerned with the appreciation of touch, pain, various movements of muscles, temperature and other sense impressions are found in the parietal lobe. The left cortex receives impulses from the right side of the body, and the right cortex from the left side of the body. If a region in the parietal cortex of the right hemisphere is destroyed, say, then there is no sensation of the left side of a person. This is due to the crossing of nerve tracts from one side of the body to another at a lower level in the central nervous system, a phenomenon known as *decussation*. The one exception to this is the pathway from the eye to the brain. There fibres from the right half of *each* eye go to the right side of the brain, and similarly fibres from the left half of each eye go to the left side of the brain. So that if the right visual cortex is destroyed, then a person becomes blind in the right half of each eye. The visual cortex lies in the occipital region, at the back of the head. As an example of the further complexity of the cortex which we have not really investigated in this section, the visual cortex is thought to be divided up into sub-areas, one dealing with visual perception (a lesion here causing blindness), one connected with visual recognition (a patient with this section destroyed may see something but not recognise what he sees or attach any meaning to it), and another sub-area having to do with the faculty of revisualisation. Destruction of this area in a patient results in an inability to revisualise scenes or persons. The auditory areas are located in the temporal lobe. In this lobe also lies the root of many curious phenomena reported by Penfield.[11] By means of electrical stimulation, a classical method for the investigation of the functions of the brain, he has been able to stimulate memories, dreams and odd hallucinations in subjects.

The region in the parietal area which we have already discussed regarding sensory impressions, lies opposite the motor cortex. These two strips are divided by a central fissure. The motor area is actually in the frontal lobe. Destruction of any part of it results in the loss of voluntary movement of the appropriate part of the

[11] Penfield, W. See for example: "The role of the temporal cortex in certain psychical phenomena. The Twenty-Ninth Maudsley Lecture". *Journal of Mental Science*, 1955, *101*, 451.

body. On the other hand electrical stimulation of some part of the motor cortex arouses movement of the appropriate part of the body. The area for vocalisation also lies in this motor strip.

Besides the sensory and motor functions, there are vast areas of the cortex which are devoted to associative functions. It is obvious that the sensory and motor functions must somehow be connected and integrated. It is also clear that the complex operations of thinking, remembering and learning call for equally complex operations in the cortical regions. The sub-areas of the visual cortex which we have already described are in effect association areas. The association areas in the frontal lobe are important for the processes of reasoning and motivation. We shall describe this aspect further below.

Complexity of the Brain. The above is a very brief outline of the functions of the cerebral cortex and other parts of the brain. The cortex is related to the older parts of the brain by means of nerve tracts. Although we have made the exposition simple and have talked of "areas" and "centres" for this and that function, it is worth while, even at the expense of confusing the reader, to emphasise that the state of affairs is far more complex than this. The immensity of the cortex is worth while considering. There are approximately about fifty thousand nerve cells per square millimetre in the surface of the convolutions.[12] While we have talked about centres, it would be more correct to state that there are relatively separate patterns of function in different areas. There are secondary areas of sensory and motor representations. As is well known in some types of paralysis, loss of movement can be regained due to the taking over of control by other regions of the brain. While there are relatively specialised areas for sensation and movement, in acts involving learning and memory, the cortex works as a whole. As Lashley[13] has formulated it, the parts of the cortex are equipotential in this respect. Lastly it must be said that different schools of physiology have differed to some extent in the degree to which they attribute different areas of the brain to functions of the body. Although the idea that there were different areas of the brain partitioned for such functions as "will" has

[12] Eccles, J. C. *The Neurophysiological Basis of Mind.* Oxford 1953.
[13] Lashley, K. S. *Brain Mechanisms and Intelligence.* Univ. of Chicago Press 1929.

long been given up, there are still some textbooks of physiology which contain elaborate charts of the brain showing areas for complex operations.

Brain Structure and Personality. Allowing for the complexity of the cortex and other regions of the brain, we are now in a position to discuss the relationship between personality and brain structures. The evidence for this relationship comes from two sources. From accidental damage to parts of the brain, whether it be from internal causes such as tumours or inflammation, or from external causes such as an automobile accident; and from operations upon the brain itself—psycho-surgery as it is called. Although other parts of the brain have influence in personality disorders, it is the frontal lobes that have been discovered to be the most relevant. The frontal areas are joined by association fibres with the thalamus and other centres in the diencephalon. It will be remembered that in this latter region lie areas of emotional function. When the frontal lobes are removed as in the operation of pre-frontal leuchotomy (the word comes from the instrument used: the leucotome. Leuchotomy refers to the case when the lobes are severed from their connections on both sides of the brain. When one side of the brain is severed the term used is lobotomy), then there is found to be an alteration in the emotional force of an animal or human. Patients who have had a very great and abnormal anxiety have had relief by this operation. There is a weakening of emotional drive. Also there is a diminution in attention. Patients who have had tumours in the upper frontal areas have shown difficulty in grasping problems, and a slowing of speech and thought. Greenblatt and Myerson[14] have summarised the effects of lobotomy upon personality under various headings. Loss of drive appears to be an aspect that usually although not always occurs. There is a lack of self concern. The patient becomes less sensitive; shyness and self-reserve dropping away. His behaviour in the social sense is less turned in, he becomes more sociable but lacks tact and diplomacy. In leuchotomy the patient's emotional life becomes more shallow and superficial. His sexual behaviour is on the whole unchanged, although there may be a lack of drive here too; it is balanced, however, inasmuch that the

[14] Greenblatt, M. and Myerson, P. G. "Psychosurgery" in Weider: *Contributions Towards Medical Psychology* Part I.

patient no longer has any inhibiting influence which an anxiety about sexual matters might bring.

It is not easy to assess with any exactitude the effect of damage or removal of areas of the brain on personality, as there is bound to be shock at the very least to the neighbouring areas. Nevertheless out of the confusion and difficulty of tracing behaviour from brain, a few significant items have emerged, which we have briefly touched. We may confidently expect important new findings on personality to come from this branch of medicine.

CONSTITUTIONAL TYPES

From the time of Hippocrates (425 B.C.) there have been numerous attempts to classify people into different physical types, and to correlate these with temperament and characteristic disease. We cannot trace all of these attempts; we can only refer to two noteworthy modern examples.

Kretschmer's Classification. The first of these is the typology of Kretschmer,[15] based mainly on clinical material. He distinguished three body types: the *asthenic*, *athletic* and *pyknic*. The asthenic has long limbs and a small trunk; the pyknic has short limbs, thick neck and a large round torso. The athletic type is intermediate, being characterised by a symmetry of limb and trunk. As has been pointed out, Kretschmer revived the Greek terms pyknic, meaning compact, and asthenic, meaning without strength, as a substitute for what in older terminologies of physique has been called macro- and micro-splanchic (large heavy bodies and short limbs, and small trunks and relatively long limbs respectively). With these types of physique Kretschmer correlated the temperaments of two main groups of people with abnormal mentality. The first of these, the manic-depressives, are people who are characterised by a cyclical fluctuation in behaviour, ranging from the deepest depression to the opposite pole of excited elation. The temperament of such patients has been labelled *"cyclothyme"*. Kretschmer found in his mental hospital population that the majority of manic-depressives had pyknic physiques; hence the correlation between cyclothyme temperament and this type of physique. With the second type of mental disease, schizophrenia (characterised by a withdrawal of interest in the world), goes the

[15] Kretschmer, E. *Physique and Character*. Kegan Paul 1925.

165

other body type—the asthenic build. The term *"schizoid"* is used to describe the respective temperament. Although Kretschmer's classification had undoubted biological intuition, it is generally accepted that his formulation lack adequate criteria and the overlapping of types has given rise to confusion.

Sheldon's Classification. The error in specifying that there are so many different kinds of people, and the difficulty of pigeon-holing intermediate types into this assumption, has been avoided by Sheldon,[16] who on a basis of many hundreds of photographs of people has maintained that there is a continuous distribution of physiques. They are graded according to the predominant component. Of components there are three, derived from layers of the embryo, called endomorphy, mesomorphy and ectomorphy. In Sheldon's own definition these are described as follows:

"Endomorphy means relative predominance of soft roundness throughout the various regions of the body. When endomorphy is dominant the digestive viscera are massive and tend relatively to dominate the bodily economy.

Mesomorphy means relative predominance of muscle, bone, and connective tissue. The mesomorphic physique is normally heavy, hard, and rectangular in outline. Bone and muscle are prominent and the skin is made thick by a heavy underlying connective tissue.

Ectomorphy means relative predominance of linearity and fragility. In proportion to his mass, the ectomorph has the greatest surface area and hence relatively the greatest sensory exposure to the outside world. Relative to his mass he also has the largest brain and central nervous system."

These components are rated in degrees from one to seven. The final result is put in the form of three successive figures referring to the above components. Thus the extreme endomorph would be represented by 711, the extreme mesomorph as 171, and the extreme ectomorph as 117. The total configuration of this measurement is known as a *"somatotype"*. In his book on physique Sheldon gives elaborate photographs and descriptions of all the possible variations.

[16] Sheldon, W. H., Stevens, S. S. and Tucker, W. B. *The Varieties of Human Physique:* and Sheldon and Stevens *The Varieties of Temperament.* Harper 1940 and 1942.

Temperament. A later investigation with similar assumptions of a continuum of traits was made into temperament. Again a three-fold component classification was derived, rated in the same manner. The individual who manifests love of comfort, relaxation, pleasure in digestive activities, sleeps deeply and has need of people when in trouble, is called a *"viscerotonic"*, called so because of the predominance of visceral functioning. The *"somatotonic"* has a love of physical adventure, is assertive of posture and movement, needs exercise, has a lust of power, liable to be over mature in appearance, has a need for action when troubled, and has a spartan indifference to pain. The *"cerebrotonic"* restrains himself in posture and movement, tends to be self conscious, secretive, has a youthful manner, and prefers solitude when troubled. Only a few of the traits are given here; in the short form of Sheldon's original scale there are thirty traits given to each type of temperament. As might be expected, the temperamental components of viscerotonia, somatotonia and cerebrotonia were found to synchronise to a high degree of correlation with the respective physiques of endomorphy, mesomorphy and ectomorphy.

In typing personality from constitutional aspects as these, there is the caution that glandular influences must be taken into account, and that a person's adaptation to his own temperament or physique is another factor to be considered.

EVALUATION

It has been found necessary to provide this long section on the biological basis of personality in order to compensate for the purely psychological and social sections that are to follow. It is often forgotten that the form and functioning of our bodies exerts a powerful influence on our personalities. Nevertheless many other important factors cannot yet be explained in the language of physiology, and need to be discussed with another terminology.

PSYCHO-ANALYTICAL ASPECTS

The psycho-analytic viewpoint of personality was evolved over a number of years from a study of neurotic and normal people. From the technique of "free association", which will be explained below, there has developed a body of theory and findings which has enriched the study of personality. As these are closely connected with the technique, it is appropriate to discuss this first.

FREE ASSOCIATION

The purpose of this method is to reveal deep tendencies within the individual which otherwise seldom come to the surface, yet which nevertheless influence his behaviour. The practice consists in placing a patient in a comfortable position, insulated from the distractions of outside impressions, in order that all his mental activity be directed to his own thoughts. Everything that passes through the patient's mind is asked to be told to the analyst, particularly those thoughts and ideas which the patient considers irrelevant or of no significance or even completely nonsensical. Embarrasing thoughts or ideas which bring painful associations are especially noted. On account of the fact that resistances tend to repress much of the possible material, the entire process may take a long time. In the course of the analysis the thoughts and memories discharged are accompanied by a high degree of emotion, a process called "abreaction". It is the goal of the free association method that the hitherto unconscious material should be made conscious, the resistance overcome and the lapses of memory made up. The essential role of this technique is at once the uncovering of unconscious wishes and thoughts together with the interpretation of the forces repressing them.

The technique of free association is not the only avenue of approach that psycho-analysis uses. In addition there is the material drawn from dreams, the study of unintentional remarks and actions, and an investigation of the patient's life history. Besides these methods, the phenomenon of transference (discussed in the previous Chapter) has provided psycho-analysis with another line of attack, one which has become of increasing importance in therapy.

THE STRUCTURE OF THE MIND

By means of the above methods, Freud[17] built up a picture of personality which he had gained from his patients.

Pleasure and Reality Principles. Central to the theory of unconscious wishes and the phenomena of repression and resistance is

[17] Freud, S. *Beyond the Pleasure Principle*, Hogarth Press, 1922; *The Ego and the Id.* Hogarth Press 1927.

the contention that man lives in a polarity of two principles, the pleasure and reality principles. The chief desire of the organism is to satisfy its basic instincts, but at the same time contrariwise develops a realisation that the demands of the external world have to be met and the desire for pleasure modified. Dream material indicates that wishes which are not fulfilled in an actual sense reappear as part of the dream content. Fantasy thinking is a persistence of thought activity which does not come under the modifications imposed by the reality principle. The interaction of these two principles arouses an inevitable conflict within the personality, which result in compromise behaviour.

The Id, Ego and Super-Ego. Around 1920 Freud constructed a theory which divided the mind into three layers, namely the Id, the Ego and the Super-Ego. Together these three parts represent the dynamic nature of the psyche.

The id is the oldest and most primitive part of the psyche. It is essentially unorganised, and contains all factors of a genetic and constitutional nature. It is the storehouse of the instincts. Its content does not reach consciousness directly, but its influence is indicated in dream symbols and in neurotic symptoms.

The ego is a development of the id which has come to serve as a link between the instinctual forces in the id and the outside world. It is mostly conscious, although not always so. It also serves as a buffer between the id and the super-ego. Apart from serving the functions of selecting stimuli in the outside world, of storing up experiences and of directing the organism in voluntary movement, the ego also acts as a controlling and directing force over the id. In other words the ego is concerned with the enforcement of the reality principle, while the id is dominated by the pleasure principle.

The third force in the structure of the psyche is the super-ego. It is formed as the result of the unconscious influence of parents and teachers in early life. By unconscious precept there is constructed an entire edifice which is concerned with moral principles and rules of conduct.

These three forces are not necessarily mutually exclusive. To a certain extent they are inter-penetrative. Their relation in behaviour is exemplified in the explanation of certain phenomena like guilt and anxiety, and self-punishment. An abnormal feeling of guilt is explained by reference to the abnormal severity of the super-ego, a code of morals laid down in childhood which the person cannot possibly live up to. Unaware of this he nevertheless feels that his particular transgression cannot ever be absolved. Anxiety is looked upon as a danger signal when repressed tendencies in the id threaten to break into the domain of the ego. The ego feels fear although it is not quite certain about what it is afraid. Self-punishment is the result of a union of id and super-ego. The aggressive tendencies, which were at first thought to originate with the id, are deflected from an outside object by the unconscious moral principles which result in the aggressive tendencies being turned against the self.

DEFENCE MECHANISMS

We have noted that anxiety is a danger signal to the ego. The danger comes from the internal systems of the psyche, namely the id and the super-ego. Conflict can develop between demands of the id and the ego, and the super-ego and the ego. In order to meet the stress caused by these conflicts, a number of mechanisms are set up which defend the ego from excessive internal attacks. These ego-defence mechanisms work by distorting reality and diverting the natural outlet of energy. Through their operation the ego is safe-guarded with a façade of illusion.

Projection. This is the case where inadmissible wishes of the self are attributed on to another. In the original form in which this term was used it is a defence mechanism of ascribing to others desires that are not admitted in oneself. Sears[18] quotes an experiment by Wright concerning this. "Eight-year-old children were given pairs of toys, one a preferred toy and one non-preferred, and then asked to give one toy to a friend to play with. Immediately afterwards they were asked which toy the friend would have given away. The proportion of times that the friend was considered generous (giving away the preferred toy) was much less after the conflict situation—in which the child himself was forced to give away a toy, than it was after a control situation in which the child did not have to give away a toy." It was concluded from this that stinginess is projected when the person feels

[18] Sears, R. R. "Experimental Analysis of Psychoanalytic Phenomena" in J. M. Hunt *Personality and the Behavior Disorders.* Vol. I.

guilty about his own stinginess. Sears himself sums it up by saying that "projection, as a defence mechanism, accompanies a lack of insight into one's own qualities and that guilt accompanying a particular kind of action can initiate the projection."

Sublimation. Here the desire for a socially disapproved object can be transferred on to an approved one. In the original formulation by Freud it was construed as a deflection of the sexual impulse from the act itself to performances of another nature. A person rejected in love transforms his erotic impulses to some creative work. Although experimental work on the nature of this mechanism has not proved altogether supporting, it must be remembered that it is a concept difficult to ascertain precisely.

Identification. Where a motive is unable to be achieved personally, satisfaction is obtained by participation in the ideals or activities of other people or groups. Thus young nurses might tend to identify themselves with Florence Nightingale, shop girls with the activities on the screen of Marilyn Monroe. The success of romantic stories in some women's magazines is due largely to this tendency. In extreme cases it can lead to the grossest illusions, as in the case of mental patients considering themselves to be Napoleon. Used in a less extreme sense it is no more than vicarious participation.

Reaction Formation. This is a concept that, by its very nature, is difficult to define in any strict manner. It pertains to the fact that if a person has a strong impulse to do (or avoid from) an action which is not approved, then he performs an act which is the very opposite. A coward, for example, performs some act of bravery. A reformed drunkard becomes a temperance lecturer, and so forth.

Repression. The best known of Freudian mechanisms concerns the banishment of intolerable ideas or wishes from the conscious fringe of behaviour to the unconscious. Here, however, although not conscious they still persist in influencing behaviour, so that a person may be said to be dominated in his actions by unconscious wishes. Experimental validation of this mechanism was demonstrated by Erikson[19] in his tests with post-hypnotic suggestion.

---

[19] Erikson, M. H. "Experimental demonstrations of the psychopathology of everyday life". *Psycho-Analytic Quarterly* 1939, *8*, 338.

In these experiments subjects were hypnotised and instructed that when they awoke they would repress particular impulses. Results showed that these instructions were carried out, although the subjects were unaware of the underlying instructions, and despite showing manifestations of uneasiness.

Regression. This idea is connected with the order of emotional development to be described below. When a person is said to have slipped back from a higher stage of emotional maturity to a lower one, it is called "regressive activity". In a naïve way we might suppose that an adult who exhibits temper tantrums can be said to have regressed from the type of behaviour appropriate to adults to a type of behaviour more appropriate in young children.

THE GENETIC PROCESS

It is one of the central theses of Freudian theory that events in the early life of an individual have a marked effect on the adult personality pattern. Connected with this is the part played by instinct in the formation of character. What is meant by the term Instinct here will be discussed first.

The Instinct Theories. Fundamental to these is the part played by what Freud termed the "libido". This concept was used in a manner as Freud himself put it of a physicist with a fluid electric current. To quote him[20] ". . . among the psychic functions there is something which should be differentiated (an amount of affect, a sum of excitation), something having all the attributes of a quantity . . . a something which is capable of increase, decrease, displacement and discharge, and which extends itself over the memory traces of an idea like an electric charge over the surface of the body." Now libido was related to the sexual instincts by being the force by which the latter are represented in the mind. The libido does not appear fully fledged at puberty; it is characterised by a steady progression from babyhood, through stages in the first five years of life, right through childhood and adolescence to the appearance of sexual functions proper. An account of the significance given to these stages represents the causal-genetic assumptions, which really incorporate what has been called

[20] Freud, S. "The Defence Neuro-Psychoses" (1894) *Collected Papers*, Vol. I. Hogarth Press 1946.

the first instinct theory. The idea of libido was applied in an explanatory manner to various neuroses. Thus in hysteria, this energy was blocked from its normal outlet and flowed into other organs, becoming fixated at certain points. This was generally associated with the theory that a person was faced with an unbearable idea, which was made innocuous by its "conversion" into some bodily form. In the case of compulsive states, the intolerable feeling was transferred to some other idea or act not associated with the original thought. Also in anxiety states, the conception of the libido was brought in with the notion of "free floating" anxiety.[21]

As already noted, Freud's first theory of the instincts was connected with the assumptions bound up with the progression of the sexual impulse in the early life of the child. The two principles that governed his viewpoint at this stage of his thought were those of self-preservation and the need for procreation. As such he centred almost exclusively on the sexual instincts. In what came to be known as the second instinct theory, Freud shifted his attention away from the sexual aspects and on to the self-preservation side. His earlier formulations failed to explain the facts of aggression. These could not explain the impulse to destructiveness which appeared to him as a basic instinct. Side by side with the emphasis on aggression there came the observation that people tended to repeat earlier actions, and to go over the same behaviour again and again during their lifetime. These new speculations resulted in a change of theory; the conception of the libido was partly given up. There was presented a basic conflict between two fundamental instincts—the life instinct (Eros) and the death instinct (Thanatos). He supposed that there was a desire for organic life to return to the inorganic state. Freud himself stated the matter in this way:[22] "We may suppose that the final aim of the destructive instinct is to reduce living things to an inorganic state. For this reason we also call it the *death instinct*. If we suppose that living things appeared later than inanimate

[21] *Hysteria* is a nervous disorder characterised by dissociation; a variety being *conversion hysteria* in which there is a paralysis of a part of the body not attributable to an organic reason. *Compulsion* is an irresistible act which the patient feels constrained to perform notwithstanding its irrational character; similarly *obsessions* refer to recurring ideas which the patient cannot get rid of, and are also irrational. Groundless apprehensions and fears are characteristic of *anxiety states*.

[22] Freud, S. *An Outline of Psycho-Analysis*. Hogarth Press 1949.

ones and arose out of them, then the death instinct agrees with the formula that we have stated, to the effect that instincts tend towards a return to an earlier state. We are unable to apply the formula to Eros (the love instinct). That would be to imply that living substance had once been a unity but had subsequently been torn apart and was now tending towards re-union. In biological functions the two basic instincts work against each other or combine with each other. Thus, the act of eating is a destruction of the object with the final aim of incorporating it, and the sexual act is an act of aggression having as its purpose the most intimate union. This interaction of the two basic instincts with and against each other gives rise to the whole variegation of the phenomena of life. The analogy of our two basic instincts extends from the region of animate things to the pair of opposing forces—attraction and repulsion—which rule in the inorganic world."[23]

Causal Genetic Assumptions. There are two main theses: the first is that of infantile sexuality. Emotional and sexual development followed a progression analogous to physical maturation. The sexual impulse did not appear suddenly at puberty with the appearance of sexual behaviour proper; there were already signs of sexuality in the young child and even as far back as babyhood. At this point it is necessary to try and see what Freud meant by "sex". It is a remarkable fact, considering all that has been written on sex from the psycho-analytic point of view that there does not exist in Freud's own writings any really clear definition of what he meant by the word. It is only obvious that he was not restricting himself to it being synonymous with "genital behaviour". What he stressed was that the baby and then the child achieved pleasure (and this was interpreted as erotic pleasure) from various regions of the body, known as erotogenic zones. During the first few years of life there were three distinct stages connected with three areas of the body. These phases were known as the oral, anal and phallic stages, and the areas of the body they were connected with were the mouth, the anus and the genitals respectively (although not with the mature functions of the last). Interest at these stages was centred on the functions of

[23] For a concise description of the two instinct theories see Thompson, C. *Psycho-Analysis: Evolution and Development.* Allen and Unwin 1952.

the three bodily areas. At the oral stage the baby is largely concerned and has pleasure with processes of nutrition and sucking. At the anal period, emphasis shifts and includes the functions of excretion and toilet training. Thirdly the child comes to realise the fact that he or she possesses sexual organs and attention is turned to these. The relations of the child with its parents then enters into a significant period which is known as the Oedipus situation. If the child is a boy there is a desire for a certain relation with his mother, a relation which Freud unequivocally called sexual. This was combined with fears of castration and hostility towards his father. If the child is a girl there develops an attachment to the father known as the Electra complex.

These early stages are followed by the latency period which brings the child to the age of puberty and the full development of sexual organs.

The second thesis is that these early stages leave a mark on the adult personality. The development of the libido over these milestones is looked upon as a necessary progression of maturation of character. If, for some reason or another, there develops any conflict at any stage with the result that the child does not live through the experiences connected with it, then the personality structure of the adult suffers accordingly. Thus the adage that the child is father to the man receives a peculiar twist. It is to be remembered that these postulates of primary stages were furnished retrospectively, that is by the interpretations given to clinical material of the free associations of patients, although confirmatory evidence was looked for in children's behaviour. The protocols of adult cases of depression showed that there was an undue interest in oral matters; in obsessional states there was an unconscious preoccupation with anal matters. Similarly hysterics showed evidence of equivalent links with the phallic stage of development. All this evidence suggested that people suffering from such mental illnesses were people who had either not grown out of an early stage of development, who had not lived completely through them, or had "regressed" to an earlier stage.

EVALUATION

We have done no more than sketch some of the major contributions of psycho-analysis to the study of personality. It is a subject which has influenced many other branches of psychology and the social sciences.[24] In relation to personality, it has placed the emphasis on mechanisms of a quasi-biological nature. As we shall see in the next section, there has been a tendency to move away from a biological emphasis to that of a more socially oriented one, yet still retaining the basic psycho-analytic approach.

It is difficult to provide an evaluation of Freudian theory which will both satisfy the ordinary requirements of scientific method and do justice to the meaningful findings of psycho-analysis. Woodworth's summary is perhaps representative of the outlook of modern psychologists: "The net result, so far, is that Freud's statements regarding child life and development are overgeneralised, to say the least, while some of his dynamic laws can be verified or paralleled in relatively simple laboratory situations. Young children do show some of the sex interest that Freud assumed (though whether it is genuine libido or a liking for what is hidden and forbidden is not so clear). Some children do pass through a phase much like Freud's Oedipus situation, though it is the exception rather than the rule. Freud's idea that the memories of early childhood are lost because of repression occurring at the close of the early sexual period seems to be pretty well disproved, and the existence of a clear cut "latency period" of sex interest in later childhood is very doubtful. On the other side of the ledger, it has been found possible to set up laboratory experiments demonstrating the tendency to *repress* and forget experiences that were humiliating to the individual, the tendency to *project* or attribute to other people those characteristics of the self which one is unwilling to admit, and the tendency when frustrated to *regress* to earlier and perhaps more infantile ways of acting. It is freely admitted that the laboratory situations are mild affairs in comparison with the emotional difficulties that sometimes entangle a person in real life. For that reason the experimenters may never succeed in putting some of Freud's dynamic principles to the test, but it is reassuring to have some of them verified in a small way and so brought down out of the clouds and made available, along with the experimenter's abundant material on the processes

---

[24] The following texts can be consulted. Brill, A. A. *The Basic Writings of Sigmund Freud.* Modern Library 1938. Munroe, R. L. *Schools of Psycho-Analytic Thought.* Dryden Press 1955. And in relation to social work, Heiman, M. *Psycho-Analysis and Social Work.* International Universities Press 1953.

of learning and perception, for incorporation into the growing science of dynamic psychology."[25]

SOCIAL ASPECTS

The individual is not only a product of the powerful biological forces operating within his own body; he is also moulded by the social influences at work during the time of his early upbringing and his later development. It is not just that a person has to conform in behaviour to society; in one manner of speaking he is a replica of that society, both being shaped by it and helping to shape it. To escape from the influences of the culture that one has been born into is only a little less than the impossibility of escaping from the influences of one's body. We have already discussed the social impact on the basic psychological processes of motives, learning, perception and communication. When we look at personality, the emphasis turns on the facets which an individual displays to his fellows as co-members of society. It is not to be suggested that there is a conscious mask presented to society. Sometimes there may be as with the characters in Ibsen's play *The Pillars of Society*; but more often than not there is a layer of the personality that has been so conjoined with its culture that it is difficult to say whether the one has created the other. And it is this layer which occupies our attention in this section. As far as attention from psychology is concerned, the last twenty years has seen a greater and greater interest in this subjèct. The effect of field studies in primitive cultures by psychologically minded anthropologists has made us realise how exactly determined people are by their social environment. And when we enquire into the more complicated nature of our own society and the groups within that, again it can be seen how the personality of man is marked by the culture and sub-cultures in which he lives.

NEO-FREUDIANISM.

Within the sphere of psycho-analysis there has been a deviancy away from the undoubtedly biological orientation of the classical

---

[25] Woodworth, R. S. *Contemporary Schools of Psychology*. Methuen 1949, Rev. Edn. The thesis that the early stages in childhood influence personality as being universal to man, has been sharply criticised by studies of cultures other than western. See especially Orlansky, H. "Infant care and personality". *Psychol. Bull.* 1949, *46*, 1.

formulations of Freud towards an approach emphasising the impact of society on the personality. Psycho-analysts such as Karen Horney, Erich Fromm and Abram Kardiner were in the forefront of this new movement.

Horney had veered from the purely libidinal and developmental aspects of Freud's views by regarding neurosis as a function of the demands which the prevailing culture makes upon its members.[26] Aggression, for example, in our own particular society is looked upon as a reflection of the competitive values endorsed by it. Neurosis is regarded as a result of the conflict brought about by the failure of the individual to adapt to the environment. Here there is a wandering away from the emphasis in Freudian doctrine of conflict between the entities of id and ego on the one hand, and ego and super-ego on the other. With this deviancy goes an insistence on the situation here and now rather than delving into childhood experiences (a position which has been taken up by other analysts). It is possible to run through the whole gamut of analytic concepts and indicate how Horney has provided an interpretation which steers clear of an explanation couched in biological or pseudo-biological terms and moves towards an explanation more in agreement with the concepts of sociology and anthropology.

Fromm also disagreed with the basic Freudian thesis of the antisocial nature of man.[27] In his book *The Fear of Freedom* Fromm wished to show that there was not a fundamental dichotomy between man and society, but that man is continually creating society as society is creating him. Man is regarded in a historical context as having freed himself from both the bondage of nature and the bondage of groups in which he had sunk his individuality. But the price of regained individuality was the feeling of isolation, insecurity and insignificance. Neurosis is therefore seen as a result of the interaction between these two tendencies. Fromm in a later paper[28] has illustrated this interaction neatly by reference to the feelings of guilt and anxiety which were aroused by the doctrines of Calvin: "It may be said that the person who is overwhelmed by a feeling of his own powerlessness and unworthiness,

[26] Horney, Karen. *The Neurotic Personality of Our Time.* 1937.
[27] Fromm, Erich, *The Fear of Freedom.* Kegan Paul 1942.
[28] "Individual and Social Origins of Neurosis" *American Sociological Review* 1944, 9, 380. Reprinted in Rose, A. M. *Mental Health and Mental Disorder.* Routledge and Kegan Paul, 1956.

by the unceasing doubt of whether he is saved or condemned to eternal punishment, who is hardly capable of any genuine joy and has made himself into the cog of a machine which he has to serve, has a severe defect. Yet this very defect was culturally patterned; it was looked upon as particularly valuable, and the individual was thus protected from the neurosis which he would have acquired in a culture where the defect would give him a feeling of profound inadequacy and isolation." This orientation towards the social origin of maladjustment has found expression with Fromm in asking such questions[29] about our present culture as: Are we Sane? Can a society be sick? The whole trend of Fromm's work, and others like him, make us enquire about the standards by which we judge mental illness, and enable us to state the subject of personality and culture as one of mutual adaptation and not as a problem of an irreconcilable duality.

It is not quite correct to say that Freud himself was unaware of the importance of cultural pressures; his books *Group Psychology and the Analysis of the Ego, Totem and Taboo,* and *Civilisation and Its Discontents,* indicate that he had an appreciation of them. His standpoint, however, did not allow the type of enquiry which Horney and Fromm have undertaken. As a result of the latter and also of those analysts with an anthropological interest, it is becoming clearer that there is developing a theory which will be equally adaptable by the social scientist as well as the psychologist.

ROLE AND STATUS

When one turns to the social aspects of an individual one inevitably turns to the part which he plays in society. The terms "role" and "status" have been coined to indicate this feature. The second term alludes roughly to the position which a person occupies in society, while the term "role" signifies the attitudes and patterns of behaviour associated with that status. As Linton has formulated it:[30] ". . . statuses are ascribed to him on the basis of his age and sex, his birth or marriage into a particular family unit, and so forth. His roles are learned on the basis of his statuses, either current or anticipated. In so far as it represents overt behavior, a role is the dynamic aspect of a status: what the

[29] *The Sane Society*. Routledge and Kegan Paul, 1956.
[30] Linton, R. "Concepts of Role and Status". In Newcomb and Hartley: *Readings in Social Psychology*.

individual has to do in order to validate his occupation of the status." Any one person may have different statuses and thus different roles. A man may have the status of father in his family, secretary in his business, and member of his club. There are two important points about these definitions. The first is that status has its correct meaning when applied in the prestige system of the community. It is the amount of deference that other people give to a position that enhances it in the community. This may vary from group to group. Thus a high position in the Freemasonry might be credited with eminence by the members of it while to an outsider it might merely be looked upon as silly. The emphasis here is on perception, and this leads on to the other point, namely that there is an expectation attached to a role. By virtue of a position in society, a type of behaviour is expected of a person holding that position, so that obligations and duties are anticipated from that person. In a society in which there is a clear differentiation of roles, a reciprocal relationship is built up between the players of different roles. A policeman is expected by members of the public and by officials to adopt a line of procedure which is in keeping with his office. Conflict in role playing does not develop unless a person no longer performs actions which are in keeping with his expected role, or unless somebody has an expectation of a role which does not correspond with the actual role.

Role-Playing in Casework. The playing of a role can have quite precise meaning in casework as exemplified by the case quoted by Goldberg,[31] where a young alcoholic found that he could not take a drug necessary for treatment of his condition. The caseworker was constrained to play the role of a strong father, insisting that the client take the tablets. Irvine,[32] in commenting on this case and discussing the subject of role-playing in casework, has noted that "It is important to recognise that the playing of even a quite authoritative role such as this can be genuine casework, provided it is dictated by the needs of the client and the situation, and not by the worker's own need to assert himself; provided also that it is a genuine expression of the worker's concern for the

[31] Goldberg, E. M. "Function and Use of Relationship in Psychiatric Social Work". *Brit. J. Psychiatric Social Work* 1953, No. 8, p. 3.
[32] Irvine, E. E. "Transference and Reality in the Casework Relationship", *Brit. J. Psychiatric Social Work*, 1956, *3*, No. 4, p. 15.

client and not of rejection. If we do not recognise such a carrying of authority as casework we are going to confuse and undermine such caseworkers as probation officers and child care workers, who must often of necessity play just such a role; it is better to admit that even the psychiatric social worker may have clients who not only need advice, but also the experience of contact with someone who is prepared to give unpalatable advice and to take full responsibility for it. These will usually be the very weak and immature clients; we shall probably agree that it is a pity to give much advice to those who are capable of thinking out their own solutions and taking responsibility for their own decisions."

It can be seen that the idea of a role, whether employed consciously as in the above case, or whether it is merely a label given to a sequence of behaviour attached to a person's position in society, can be a useful concept so long as it does not become too generalised. There has been a tendency for the idea to be used so vaguely that it ceases to mean very little.

THE BASIC PERSONALITY

Every individual may be a unique personality, yet the study of different cultures indicates that although there is diversity, there appears also to be uniformity, at least within any one culture. This is partly a result of the fact that there are definite positions in society with their respective roles, and in the playing of these roles there is bound to be a consistency of characteristics. The fact that people from the same culture seem to possess some property in common has given rise to terms such as the "basic personality structure", "representative personality", "modal personality", and more recently "national character". These terms all point to the idea that within a society there is a common framework of traits which are shared by all the members. The term "basic personality" was first used by Kardiner;[33] it arose out of the union between anthropology and psycho-analysis. We have already discussed the traditional psycho-analytic notion of the effect of the early formative years on the later adult personality pattern, and we have also remarked upon the objections to this from the point of view of the evidence from studies of different cultures than our own. The idea of a basic personality appears as

[33] Kardiner, A. and others. *The Psychological Frontiers of Society*. Columbia University Press 1945.

a synthesis of the opposing theses. It takes notice of the fact that practices of child-rearing have influence on the adult personality, but allows that the different traits of personality are culturally and not universally determined.

The fact that a large segment of our personality pattern has this cultural background is not just a matter of theoretical interest. Sandi[34] has indicated how a knowledge of the cultural factors involved is a necessity in social work generally. He notices the trend to the "psycho-cultural" approach in social work and remarks that "in this approach towards the understanding of the individual, there is full recognition of the impact of that process by which the individual, starting through the parent-child relationship, is 'culturalised' along the lines of the persistent traditional patterns of the group".

The basic personality thesis has another important point. Namely that the constellation of attitudes and behaviour within it are those that are most conducive to the norms of the institutions of any particular society. Thus the standard set by tradition places a premium on the type of personality that fits in best with it, inasmuch that as a person wanders away from the "basic" personality he also ceases to fit in with his fellow members and hence he will tend to suffer the ensuing lack of security which society undoubtedly provides him.

It is to be further noted that while the idea of a basic personality peculiar to a culture is an important move towards the total picture of personality, and while it is useful as a model for investigations of personality, it must be remembered that it had its genesis in societies where there is a relatively homogeneous system of child rearing. In Western society there are different methods of child-rearing within the total culture,[35] and in order to establish a model of a personality, the different methods would have to be taken into account, and it is very probable that we should find more than one "basic" personality. Nevertheless, allowing for the complexity of out Western life, the idea does enable us to search for uniformities within the manifold differences

[34] Sandi, P. L. "A Cultural Approach to Social Work". *Human Organisation*, 1949, *8*, 15, Spring.
[35] The point made by Jahoda, M. "Toward a Social Psychology of Mental Health" in Rose: *Mental Health and Mental Disorder*. For a description of basic personality types in sub-cultures of our own society see Spinley, B. M. *The Deprived and the Privileged*. Routledge and Kegan Paul, 1953.

of individuals and allows the pattern of the values of society to be taken into full account.

INTELLIGENCE

The modern conception of intelligence has descended from various strands of thought—philosophical, physiological and biological, as well as from individual psychology.[36] The term itself was coined by Cicero from the Greek of Aristotle, in which he had distinguished the cognitive or intellectual aspects of the mind from the emotional and moral. At a more recent point on the spiral of history, however, it was the English philosopher Herbert Spencer who revived the term and used it to designate the important function of the organism of adaptation to the environment. In animals this may cover the relevant behaviour necessary for the acquisition of food and shelter, but in man the adaptation to his environment goes far beyond this, including such matters as the capacity to deal with mathematical symbols and the ability to manage social relationships. Modern formulations of intelligence include such definitions as "the capacity for flexible adjustment", "the ability to carry on abstract thinking", and "the ability of the individual to adjust to new problems and conditions of life". It would be correct to state that there is no clear agreement as to the nature of intelligence; that in fact, as Sprott has pointed out,[37] it is misleading even to ask such a question as "What is intelligence?" as it would seem to suggest that intelligence is something similar to an organ of the body and is tucked away in some corner of the brain.

At the present time, notwithstanding the different schools of thought on the subject, intelligence would appear to be a *general* cognitive process which is innate, and which manifests itself in the ability to perceive and deduce relationships between phenomena. Possibly a useful definition as any is that suggested by Knight:[38] "Intelligence is the ability, when we have some aim or question in mind, (a) to discover the relevant qualities and relations of the objects or ideas that are before us, and (b) to evoke

[36] Burt, Sir Cyril "The Evidence for the Concept of Intelligence". *Brit. J. Educ. Psychol.* 1955, 25, 158.

[37] Sprott, W. J. H. *Social Psychology*, Methuen 1952.

[38] Knight, R. *Intelligence and Intelligence Tests*. Methuen 1950.

other relevant ideas. In other words, it is the capacity for relational, constructive thinking, directed to the attainment of some end. The man of high intelligence is one who, faced with a problem, can seize upon the significant aspects of the objects or ideas before him, and can bring to mind other ideas that are relevant."

The statement that intelligence is a general capacity needs further qualification. There is a school of thought, originating with Charles Spearman,[39] based on experimental researches and statistical techniques, which maintains that intelligence is a compendious term for a number of factors which can be correlated but not totalled. Thus there is a factor of perceptual abilities, of numerical abilities, of verbal relations, of memory and so forth, each of which is relatively independent of the rest. But only relatively; for it has been found that there was a general ability running through all the factors. Spearman had shown by mathematical demonstration, that there were in any cognitive ability two fundamental factors: namely a general factor, which he designated simply as g, and a special ability s. Following this trend, it has been found that the common quality g tends to be manifested most in tests that are composed of items involving reasoning, and least in memory and spatial tests.

We might therefore expect that a person who can solve geometrical problems accurately will also be good at logical exercises, but that a person who can retain whole pages of Horace in his head will not necessarily be proficient at algebra.

TESTS

Since intelligence tests are the sole means that we know of indicating how intelligence works, we must now turn to their nature. At the outset it should be stressed that there is no exact science of intelligence of which the tests are an application. The tests themselves are technological devices, which are being continually refined, and which work in a more or less rough and ready manner. By means of them we can divide the bright boy from the dullard, and can grade pretty accurately the individuals lying between these two extremes. That the intelligence test has garnered in its history a store of discredit from some people, is due partly to the reason that it has often been put forward as some omniscient

[39] See Eysenck, H. J. *Uses and Abuses of Psychology.* Penguin Books, 1953, for a recent exposition.

dividing rod. The concept of "I.Q." has been invoked as an absolute value, whereas its genesis shows that it is essentially relative. The intelligence quotient is not similar to the basic metabolic rate or the amount of sugar in the blood, to quote two known constants from medicine. There is no absolute standard of intelligence in this way, common to man as a species. The I.Q. can only be measured relative to a particular test within a certain population; if it is applied to a number of tests, then the tests themselves must first be shown to have some measure of agreement.

"*I.Q.*" The intelligence quotient is defined by the simple ratio of mental age to chronological age, multiplied by one hundred. The first term is defined in its turn by giving a graded series of tests, increasing in difficulty, to a number of children differing in age. By such means it can be found that some tests can be done successfully by the majority of eight-year-old children, but not by six-year-olds. Again there are tests of further difficulty which most ten-year-old children can do, but not eight- or nine-year-old children, and so forth. Now if a child can do questions which ten-year-old children can do, then he is allotted the "mental age" of ten, whatsoever his actual age in years. If he happens to be ten years old, then his intelligence quotient will be ten divided by ten (mental age divided by chronological age), multiplied by one hundred, which equals one hundred, the defining average. If on the other hand he is only eight years old, and yet can do the tests which ten-year-old children can do, then his I.Q. would be 10/8 × 100, which is 125. In other words, he would be well above average, the term average here being the statistical mean, and not to be confused with the overtones usually given to the term "normal". Generality can be given to the I.Q. as it is known that the distribution of intelligence in the general population follows what statisticians call the normal curve of probability. That is to say, taking a random number of children and one which is large, in the order of thousands, it would be found that the I.Q.s around the defined mean of 100 would be the most frequent, while very high and very low I.Q.s would be the least frequent. Although, therefore, an I.Q. of a certain number can be given some definite interpretation, it is to be noted that the concept is only meaningful with children and adolescents to the point where intelligence tests indicate that there is a maximum of intelligence (the range differing according to the test used, but about sixteen to nineteen), after which point the tests show that there is a gradual decline. A more satisfactory method of comparing intelligence scores is to relate the findings of the same test with similar groups, within the same age range. One test, for example, can establish norms for people with grammar school education of varying ages. The same test can also be applied to university graduates and norms be established for them. Therefore any new individual who takes this test can then be compared within the limits of his own educational background. There need be no question here of the I.Q. concept; the norms are defined in the terms of the individual scores of the particular test.

Types of Tests. Intelligence tests can be classified according to whether they are verbal or non-verbal, whether they can be applied to a group or only individually. Some tests are specially designed for certain age classes, special infant tests for example, others can be given to individuals over a wide range of years. As far as their application is concerned, it is becoming more and more clear that to give one test alone is only to gain an indication. Complete reliability is only assured when a battery of tests is given. We cannot here deal with the types of tests now in use, individually. The student is referred to the references below for this;[40] we can only deal with tests in general. To that end it can be pointed out that a representative test as the Stanford-Binet (Revised Version) consists of a number of sub-tests, each appropriate to certain age levels. The content of the tests range from simple manipulation of objects to abstract reasoning, appropriate to very small children and to adults respectively. For young children the items in a test consist of placing forms in holes, identifying objects and parts of the body by pointing when they are named, building a tower and naming common objects in a picture. For an adult there are items consisting of arithmetical reasoning, vocabulary questions, reasoning tests of ingenuity, and indicating the meaning of proverbs. Other tests, such as Ravens Progressive Matrices, commonly used by the Services, consist

[40] The books by Knight and Eysenck, already quoted, are recommended. For a fuller account of testing in general see Anastasi, A.: *Psychological Testing*. MacMillan 1954.

of a number of coloured patterns from which one has to choose to fit one large pattern in which there is a section missing. In this test there is a large emphasis on perceptual ability to mark relationships; perception and deductive reasoning go hand in hand.

SOCIAL INFLUENCES

It has been stated that intelligence is an innate process; but we should supplement this by the qualification that there has been and still is some controversy about how much we should attribute to heredity and how much to environment. We shall return to this in the next section. At this point it can be said that there are a number of cultural and social factors that do influence a person's intelligence as defined and measured by an intelligence test.

Parental Occupation. One such factor is the occupation of parents in relation to the intelligence score of the child. The evidence[41] on this score points to the fact that the children of professional parents have higher intelligence quotients than the children of labourers, to quote the two extremes. It is possible to run through the gamut of occupations, from professional and semi-professional occupations, through clerical, skilled and semi-skilled trades, to slightly skilled and labourers proper, and find this sequence positively correlated with intelligence scores. When the standard of socio-economic status is used there is again found a positive correlation inasmuch as Goodenough[42] points out, that a higher percentage of bright children come from families of superior socio-economic status, while a higher percentage of children who are backward come from the lower social classes. This does not mean, of course, that there are not dull children in the higher social classes or bright children in the poorer; the assessment deals only in frequencies. The relationship with occupational and class memberships can be partly accounted for by the fact that children whose parents are in the higher income brackets are obviously provided with a better intellectual and cultural environment, which will include better education, plenty of books and in fact all those amenities which will draw out intelligence.

[41] Knight, R. *op. cit.*
[42] Goodenough, F. L. "The Measurement of mental growth in childhood". In Carmichael, L. *Manual of Child Psychology.* Wiley 1946.

Delinquency and Intelligence. Reference to such social factors has marked relevance to the question of whether delinquents have low intelligence. As has been pointed out in a pamphlet on the subject,[43] the fact that delinquents tend to be drawn to a very large extent from the lower occupational classes and from families of limited education and low cultural level, unless an allowance is made for the fact that there is to be found lower intelligence on the whole in these groups, it will be concluded that there is a correlation between low intelligence and delinquency. The importance of this allowance for the question can be seen from the author's conclusion that "The same cultural factors which depress the intelligence test score are also associated with delinquency. No enquiry in which the cultural factors common to both low test scores and delinquency have been partially controlled is conclusive. Hence the question of the relation or not of low intelligence to delinquency has not been settled."

Intelligence and Family Size. Another social factor which has given rise to a certain amount of controversy in recent years is that of the relationship between intelligence and family size. A large body of evidence has accumulated to indicate that larger families appear to produce on the whole lower intelligences (as measured by tests) than smaller families.[44] The inverse relationship is not much—the statistical correlation is about the order of —·20 to —·25, but it has been found to be fairly persistent. The reason for this inverse relationship is not known. The problem has become a point of disagreement between those who ascribe the relationship to reasons of heredity and those who maintain that it is due to conditions of environment. Actually, as Anastasi[45] makes quite clear, there are three possible explanations, which may operate as a combination of two or all three. The first is straightforward heredity; there is an inherited structural factor which limits intellectual development and which is passed on from parents to children. It follows then that "the obtained correlations would then result from the fact that, within a given

---

[43] Woodward, Mary. *Low Intelligence and Delinquency,* 1955. I.S.T.D.

[44] For contrasting views on the phenomenon see Blackburn, J. "Family Size, Intelligence Score and Social Class" and Burt, Sir Cyril "Family Size, Intelligence and Social Class". *Population Studies,* 1947, *1,* 165–186.

[45] Anastasi, A. "Tested Intelligence and Family Size" *Eugenics Quarterly* 1954, *1,* 155.

culture, persons with inferior heredity tended to have more off-spring". The second explanation is straightforward environmental; psychological differences of a motivational and emotional nature stimulating to intelligence would represent different "intellectual environments"; "in this case, the correlations between family size and intelligence of offspring would again result from a tendency for the less intelligent parents to have more children, but heredity would not be involved." The third explanation is partly economical and partly psychological. Economical in the obvious sense that large families are debarred from educative amenities (especially in the poorer classes) that smaller families might have; psychological as far as verbal ability is concerned, as it is well known that contact with adults promotes verbalization, and it is assumed that in large families there would be more contact with the other children and less with the parents.

Other Environmental Factors. We shall return later to the question of heredity, but whatsoever the outcome of the relative importance of genetic influences and environmental factors, there are a number of items included within the latter that call for attention. Blackburn[46] has summarised these in a pamphlet entitled *"Influence of the Social Environment on Intelligence Test Scores"*. He enumerates a number of factors that affect intelligence as measured by test scores, factors that include language; the attitude towards the test and competition (very different if we contrast Western society with less centralised and more primitive cultures); the emphasis on abstraction—again very prevalent in our own society; the appropriateness of the actual test given to certain groups (Blackburn cites the case of the Binet test given to canal boat children where another type of test would have been more appropriate); and finally the question of standardisation. The author points out that "it is always more meaningful to compare Tommy Jones of Camberwell with others boys of his age and social and economic class in the same district than it is to compare him with a 'representative' child of his age in the whole of Britain."

Coaching. Coaching children in the performance of intelligence tests is one further factor that might be included under the present

[46] *British Social Hygiene Council Publication* Occasional Papers, No. 4.

heading. Vernon[47] has examined the evidence on this score and indicated that although the effects of practice with intelligence tests are negligible, the effects of systematic coaching are more serious. Specifically it has been shown that the combination of coaching and practice can lead to an average increase in I.Q. of nine points. The effect is seen more with bright children than with the dull ones.

We shall reserve the evidence for the heriditary contribution of intelligence for the next section, but it is quite apparent that as far as scores on intelligence tests are concerned the diverse conditions connected with the environment have some potency.

Intelligence and Social Problems. Questions regarding intelligence loom large in the practical questions with which social science is concerned. We have already noticed its connection with delinquency, although the presence of other factors renders any connection here difficult to assess. That intelligence has further practical ramifications is brought out by a study on childbearing.[48] It was found that intelligence test scores (Raven's Progressive Matrices was used) was helpful in distinguishing those women who held a better preparatory attitude towards childbirth from others. More specifically it was seen that the use of birth control methods, the quality of diet and sources of information generally about childbearing was positively associated with intelligence. Another problem, this time relating to difficulties of behaviour, is raised by the questions formulated by Levy,[49] namely "Does a rich, dull child have problems which are characteristic of the intelligence level or the economic level of his group? Does the poor, bright child behave accordingly to those patterns which are characteristic of his economic level or of his intellectual level?" In other words there are occasions when there are two forces acting on someone at the same time—in this case intelligence and economic level—and it might be asked which force is the stronger in shaping behaviour. The conclusions drawn from this particular study were

[47] Vernon, P. E. "Symposium on the Effects of Coaching and Practice in Intelligence Tests: V. Conclusions". *Brit. J. Educational Psychol.* 1954, *24*, 57.
[48] Baird, D. and Scott, E. M. "Intelligence and Childbearing". *Eugenics Review* 1953/4, *45*, 139.
[49] Levy, J. "A Quantitative Study of the Relationship between intelligence and economic status as factors in the etiology of children's behaviour problems". *Amer. J. Orthopsychiatry* 1931, *I*, 152.

made from seven hundred case histories at the Institute for Juvenile Research at Chicago, with an age range of children from three to eighteen, two thirds of whom were boys. One of the major findings was that as intelligence increases so does the percentage of personality and emotional problems. As regards the question of social class, this study indicated that the higher social classes have personality problems, while lower social classes have social problems. What is perhaps not so expected was that the most intelligent children have the highest amount of physiological disharmonies. Sexual problems were unrelated to intelligence altogether.

CONCLUSION

In conclusion it can be said that there is little doubt that whatever is meant by the term "intelligence" there is something operating which demarcates this person from that person in the way that he adjusts himself in life, and that this ability or lack of ability enters into a great many spheres of interest for the social worker. It may be difficult to try to educe causal relationships between intelligence with this or that phenomena or behaviour, yet nothing is lost by adding to our knowledge of the other relevant variables the standards by which we have come to rate intelligence. The sole drawback arises when the concept of the I.Q. is extrapolated from its context and from the other factors of influence, and applied in a manner that is too generalised for a specific occasion.

HEREDITY AND ENVIRONMENT

Although the mechanism of heredity was not discovered until the last thirty years of the last century (and then unnoticed by the world at large until the pioneer work of Mendel was rediscovered by other investigators in 1900) the work of Darwin and his school had stressed the importance of heredity in evolution and had underlined the continuity of life. Even before Darwin, isolated thinkers had pondered over the observed fact that children appeared to have some of the traits of their parents. Leonardo da Vinci had noticed that in Ethiopia the skin colour of the inhabitants could not be attributed to the sun, as black father and black mother begat black children, but a black father and a white

mother had grey children. The mechanism of heredity is contained in every cell of the body, but particularly in the repro-
ductive cells. A cell is composed of a nucleus surrounded by a
living substance known as cytoplasm. Within the nucleus are
small bodies known as *chromosomes* which carry the hereditary
factors called genes. We need not go into the complexities of
genetics beyond this point,[50] except to repeat the familiar facts
that an individual inherits forty-eight chromosomes, half from
his father and half from his mother. Arranged in a linear order
along the chromosomes are the genes, which operate in pairs and
which together influence the development of some aspect of the
body. If both the genes are identical, then the trait which they
operate (for example curly hair) will be transmitted as such with
certainty. But if there is a gene for straight hair and a gene for
curly hair, then only one will be operative. This latter, in genetic
terminology, is called *dominant*, and the gene which does not manifest is called a *recessive*. A set of two further terms which is necessary for further discussion, are the words *genotype* and *phenotype*.
The genotype is the heredity that is received by an organism, and
the appearance of the organism is called its phenotype. Two or
more different phenotypes may have the same genotype, and
similar phenotypes may have different genotypes.

Having touched on the terms used in genetics, we can now
approach the question as to what is meant by heredity and environment. At the outset it has to be said that a great deal of what
has been discussed in the past about this topic is beside the point.
The two terms cannot be thought of as two independent unities,
as we never meet one without the other. As one noted geneticist
has said:[51] "The question whether the genotype or the environment is more important in the formation of the phenotype or the
personality is evidently meaningless (although frequently and
acrimoniously discussed). The phenotype is the outcome of a
process of organic development. There is no organic development
without an organism, and no organism without a genotype.
Equally, every organism exists in an environment and at the expense of an environment . . . any organism is the product of
its genotype and of its life experience or biography." Moreover,
at what stage does the "environment" begin? For the cytoplasm

[50] An accessible book on the subject is Kalmus H.: *Genetics*. Penguin Books 1948.
[51] Dobzhansky, T. *Evolution, Genetics and Man*. Wiley 1955.

around the nucleus in the cell is environment for the latter, and the chemical nature of this is no less important for the future development of the individual.

Interaction. It will therefore be a better usage of terms to talk about the interaction of heredity and environment, rather than the contribution of each to this or that behaviour. In this way it is more appropriate to talk of suitable or non-suitable environments for this or that genotype. For example the genotype of an albino results in a lack of the protective pigment which shields the individual from intense sunshine. Hence it can be said that areas in which there is intense sunlight are not suitable environments for this kind of person. Continuing this line of thought, it might be argued that if it can be demonstrated that there is a genetic basis for temperament, a disposition for excitability, then there would be environments which might give rise to excitability, which would then be clearly unsuitable for this type of person. But given another environment altogether, the genetic weakness may never arise, just as in hereditary diabetes ill health does not arise if there is a constant supply of insulin. Furthermore, as Anastasi remarks,[52] the terms heredity and environment are abstractions: "Each covers a multiplicity of factors which interact with each other. It is not enough to conclude that 'Environment' caused a particular behavior deviation. We must know what specific factors in the environment brought it about. Similarly, when we attribute a given behavioral characteristic to 'Heredity', we have not solved the problem; we have only formulated a problem. We must find out *what* is inherited. What is the hereditary condition which ultimately and indirectly leads to this behavior deviation, and how does it operate in bringing about the behavior under consideration?"

Now the genetics of those aspects of behaviour most relevant to the psychologist are not so well established as in much biological phenomena. By this is meant that the laws of Mendelian inheritance can be traced with more or less a high degree of accuracy with respect to such traits as albinism, eye colour, the

[52] Anastasi, Anne. "The Inherited and Acquired Components of Behavior". In *Genetics and the Inheritance of Integrated Neurological and Psychiatric Patterns*. Vol. 33, Proceedings of the Association for Research in Nervous and Mental disease. Williams and Wilkins 1954.

capacity for tasting a certain chemical, and for a certain type of idiocy. But for matters concerning temperament and intelligence, we have little knowledge of the actual genes at work. It is only by inferential means such as selective breeding and the study of pedigrees and an examination of identical twins that we can observe the working of heredity. For a discussion of heredity from this approach we must now turn to mental illness and later to intelligence.

HEREDITY AND MENTAL ILLNESS

As a preliminary to the observations made on human families and the inferences drawn from them, it is possible to cite animal studies in which it has been shown that some temperamental strains can be bred.[53] Two different strains of rats, for example, can be bred true for emotionality on the one hand and non-emotionality on the other. Aggressiveness in rats and mice was similarly found to be genetically determined. Now with humans of course we cannot selectively breed for this or that trait, but we can observe families as for example in the case of parent and child pairs, and brother and sister pairs. Straightforward temperamental differences, as in the case with the animal material, is difficult to determine genetically. Personality differences can better be seen with abnormal material, with genetic differences in mental disease. Where there has been a large scale investigation, using as an index the degree to which members of the family are genetically related (the degree ranging from relationships of half brothers or sisters, to full siblings or fraternal twins, to the cases of identical twins in which both children come from the same egg and thus have exactly similar genetic endowment) then the expectancy of psychosis is shown to be heavily dependent upon hereditary mechanisms. Kallman's study,[54] doing exactly this, indicates the expectancy of such mental diseases as schizophrenia, manic depression and involutional psychosis. To take the first as an example. This is a disease which is marked by a withdrawal of interest in the world, by dissociated thought processes, by a disintegration of the usual stable personality structure. The onset of the disease is likely to be gradual

[53] Hall, Calvin S. "The Genetics of Behavior" in Stevens: *Handbook of Experimental Psychology*.

[54] Kallman, F. J. "Genetic Aspects of Psychoses" in *Biology of Mental Health and Disease*.

and may not be readily apparent in its early stages, and it may be precipitated by a shock or strong difficulty. There are different types of schizophrenia and the symptoms may range from a gradual withdrawal from society to the strongest delusions and stages of excitement. When it is said that schizophrenia depends to a large extent on heredity, it is meant that there are some genetic mechanisms which create a temperamental disposition which is liable to the type of breakdown that is labelled schizophrenia. The exact nature of the mechanism is not known nor is it suggested that environmental influences do not play a large part in causing a breakdown. Here again is observed the interaction of heredity and environment. But to return to Kallman's findings.

On the basis of large scale observations, the expectancy of schizophrenia in the children of two normal parents is very low, ·9. In psychotic families, when we come to half-siblings, the expectancy is higher, 7·1. Among fraternal twins it is higher still, 14·5 and among identical twins it is very large indeed, 86·2. A similar tendency can be seen with the other types of psychosis mentioned, manic-depression and involutional psychosis.

From the point of view of personality, these figures are very suggestive, but it must be remembered that a disease entity consists of a number of temperamental traits. In order for a proper assessment to be made of the genetic basis of personality, the particular ingredients of personality need to be carefully distinguished. It is fitting to close this brief discussion of the contribution of genetics to personality with the words of another geneticist:[55] "Personality is a complex attribute of man, not easily reducible to a form suitable for genetical investigation. Animal genetics deals primarily with definite qualitative and quantitative differences between members of the same species. Since human genetics is analogous to animal genetics, it is most efficiently advanced by the study of well-defined characters. . . . Many of the elements out of which personality is built are suitable for genetic analysis, especially those which are associated with rare physical defects. As the concept of total personality is approached, exact measurement or precise description becomes difficult."

[55] Penrose, L. S. "Heredity". In J. M. Hunt: *Personality and the Behavior Disorders.* Vol. I.

HEREDITY AND INTELLIGENCE

The nature-nurture controversy, insofar as it affects intelligence, has centred around three fields of interest. Namely group differences, whether they be class, national or racial; orphan and foster children; and the study of identical twins.

Group Differences. Investigations of large groups have been concerned to show the innate comparisons of different populations, yet as Vernon has pointed out,[56] it is doubtful whether such studies can tell us much about heredity, as apart from the fact that it is extremely difficult to construct an intelligence test free from cultural and environmental influences, there is the fact that genetic population differences are so small that they would be covered over by even a minor cultural difference. Hence it is better to focus attention on the two remaining fields, foster children and identical twins.

Foster Children. The intelligence of foster children would tell us something about the nature of heredity as the correlation of foster children to their parents' intelligences can be calculated in comparison to control groups of children with their real parents. When this was done by Burks[57] the emphasis came down heavily on the side of inheritance as there was a far greater correlation between child and real parent than between foster child and foster parent. This does not mean that the environment is not of importance, for it has been demonstrated[58] that in the case of foster children living in Chicago, children who were sent to better educated parents in richer homes had higher intelligence quotients after four years in the foster home than those children who had been sent to poorer homes. Again we see the interactive effect of heredity and environment which is so difficult to disentangle.

Identical Twins. The evidence drawn from studies comparing

[56] Vernon, P. E. "Use of Intelligence Tests in Population Studies". *Eugenics Quarterly* 1954, *1*, 221.
[57] Burks, R. S. "The Relative Influence of Nature and Nurture upon mental development. *Nat. Soc. Stud. Educ.* 1928. *Twenty-Seventh Year Book.*
[58] Freeman, F. N., Holzinger, K. S. and Mitchell, B. C. "The influence of Environment on the Intelligence, School Achievement and Contact of Foster Children". *Twenty-Seventh Year Book.* This and the previous reference have been included to make the point that evidence can always be found for both sides of the nature-nurture controversy. For more factual information see "Intelligence: Its nature and nurture". *Nat. Soc. Stud. Educ.* 1940. *Thirty-Ninth Year Book.* Parts I and II.

the intelligences within a family on a sliding scale from identical twins to children who are cousins shows unmistakably the operation of genetic factors, as the correlation of identical twins in a typical study is around the order of ·9 while that of ordinary brother and sister is around ·5 and cousins are ·27. There is no correlation at all between unrelated children. Yet it is possible to find that there is quite a large difference in correlation of intelligence between identical twins who have been reared together and those that have been reared apart. This is no real contradiction; it merely means that we have to give up the notion of regarding this controversy as being composed of two antithetical elements which we can assess in an additive manner.

Statements like "intelligence is due to such and such percent of heredity and such and such percent of environment" are misleading. Anastasi and Foley present a hypothetical case concerning identical twins in separate foster homes:[59]

"Suppose we find a 10-point difference in I.Q. between two identical twins reared in separate foster homes, and a 30-point difference in I.Q. between two unrelated children reared in the same two foster homes as the twins. Can we argue that the 10-point difference between the identical twins measures the 'differentiating effect' of these two home environments, and can we therefore analyse the 30-point difference between the unrelated children into 10 points attributable to environment and 20 points attributable to heredity? Could we conclude that, insofar as these cases show, heredity was twice as important as environment in the production of individual differences in I.Q.? If we follow the concept of interaction, the answer to both questions is "No". Actually, a very slight hereditary difference between the two unrelated children may have greatly augmented the difference between the effective environments of the two foster homes, i.e. between the active stimulus-value of the environments of the two unrelated children. The effective environmental difference between the two homes would thus have been much greater for the unrelated children than for the identical twins. No simple subtraction of the end-products could disentangle the relative contribution of the factors whose initial interaction led to the obtained difference in I.Q."

[59] Anastasi, A. and Foley, J. P. "A proposed re-orientation in the heredity-environment controversy". *Psychol. Review* 1948, *55*, 239.

Evaluation. Heredity by itself as it affects intelligence only has meaning in the case of mental defectives in which it has been shown that the deficiency can be attributed to some known genetic defect. But in the more general cases we can only say that what has been transmitted to us by nature depends for its development upon nurture. Intelligence being a general term, it remains to be discovered the specific features that are embraced by that term and to see whether these are genetically transmitted, and if they are, then what type of environment helps them to develop best, or conversely what type of environment does not assist them. And in exactly the same way that we would not advise a sunny environment for the albino, so might there be advice for intellectual traits. Whether or not this will ever come about depends upon further research.

All life is an interplay between heredity and environment. In man their interaction pervades his bodily and psychological processes. All that has been discussed in this book under the five-fold scheme of Motivation, Learning, Perception, Communication and Personality, can be regarded as aspects of the total psychological apparatus effected by this interaction.

INDEX

199

Index

Stern, W., 130, 132, 133–134
Stevens, S. S., 166n.
Stratton, G. M., 85n.
Sturt, M., 96n.
Sublimation, 171
Suggestion, 86
Sullivan, H. S., 148n.
Super-ego, 169–170

Taft, R., 114
Tagiuri, R., 113, 114
Taylor, C., 101
Taylor, J. G., 83n.
Temperament, 150, 165, 167
Testimony, 125–135
Thompson, C., 174n.
Thorndike, E. L., 50–51
Thouless, R. H., 82
Thurstone, L., 64
Trait, 151
Transference, 146–148
Trial and error, 50–51
Tucker, W. B., 166n.
Turner, R., 40
Type, 151

Unemployment, 40–41

Values, 22–28
  and delinquency, 26–27
  and interests, 24–25
  breakdown of, 37
  cultural diversity of, 25–27
  peer group, 27–28
Verin, O., 69n.
Vernon, M., 81n.
Vernon, P. E., 23, 24, 190, 196
Vickery, K., 126n.
Vinacke, W. E., 98n.
Vitamins, 160
Volkart, E. H., 72, 78

Walter, A. A., 119n.
Way, Lewis, 17n.
Wertheimer, M., 81
Wilder, R. M., 160n.
Williams, J. J. B., 140n.
Witmer, H. L., 33n.
Wolff, W., 103
Wolters, A. W. P., 126n., 129, 134
Woodward, M., 188n.
Woodworth, R. S., 145, 177
Würzburg school, 4

Zuni indians, 25–26